Interprofessional Rehabilitation

A Person-Centred Approach

Edited by

Sarah G. Dean
Senior Lecturer in Health Services Research,
University of Exeter Medical School, United Kingdom

Richard J. Siegert
Professor of Psychology and Rehabilitation,
School of Rehabilitation and Occupation Studies
and School of Public Health and Psychosocial Studies,
AUT University, Auckland, New Zealand

William J. Taylor
Associate Professor in Rehabilitation Medicine,
Rehabilitation Teaching and Research Unit,
University of Otago Wellington, New Zealand

WILEY-BLACKWELL

A John Wiley & Sons, Ltd., Publication

Library of Congress Cataloging-in-Publication Data

Interprofessional rehabilitation : a person-centred approach / edited by Sarah G. Dean, Richard J. Siegert, William J. Taylor.
        p. ; cm.
    Includes bibliographical references and index.
    ISBN 978-0-470-65596-2 (pbk. : alk. paper)
    I. Dean, Sarah G.   II. Siegert, Richard J.   III. Taylor, William J., 1964–
    [DNLM: 1. Rehabilitation–psychology.   2. Evidence-Based Medicine.   3. Patient Care Team.
4. Treatment Outcome.   WB 320]
    616.86′03–dc23
                                                        2012015864

A catalogue record for this book is available from the British Library.

Wiley also publishes its books in a variety of electronic formats. Some content that appears in print may not be available in electronic books.

Cover design by Meaden Creative
Cover image © iStock

Set in 10.5/12.5pt Times by SPi Publisher Services, Pondicherry, India
Printed in Singapore by Ho Printing Singapore Pte Ltd

1   2012

Contents

About the editors

Sarah G. Dean, PhD, CPsychol, MSc, MCSP, Grad Dip Phys, BSc Jt Hons, Senior Lecturer in Health Services Research, part of the Peninsula Collaboration for Leadership in Applied Health Research and Care (PenCLAHRC) based at the University of Exeter Medical School, United Kingdom. Sarah is a chartered physiotherapist who trained at Guy's Hospital London, after completing her first degree in psychology and physical education at the University of Birmingham, United Kingdom. She worked clinically in both the NHS and private sector, specializing in musculoskeletal rehabilitation, particularly exercise therapy for sports injuries and cardiac rehabilitation. During this time she was competing as an athlete representing Great Britain in the 400 m hurdles. From 1995 she lectured in physiotherapy for nearly nine years at the University of Southampton and completed her PhD in health psychology in 2003. Her PhD investigated the use of illness perceptions for facilitating adherence to physiotherapy exercises for people with low back pain. In 2004 Sarah went to work in New Zealand as a senior lecturer in rehabilitation at the University of Otago, Wellington as part of the interprofessional Rehabilitation Teaching and Research Unit, she became a chartered psychologist in 2006. In 2009 Sarah returned to the United Kingdom to take up her current post. Sarah's research interests include applying psychology to rehabilitation medicine, such as goal setting and facilitating adherence to exercise therapy, for a number of different chronic conditions including stroke, low back pain and urinary incontinence. She uses qualitative and mixed methods for her research. Sarah teaches undergraduate medical students and supervises postgraduate students.

Richard J. Siegert, BSc, MSocSci, PGDipPsych(Clin), PhD, Professor of Psychology and Rehabilitation, School of Rehabilitation and Occupation Studies and School of Public Health and Psychosocial Studies, AUT University, Auckland, New Zealand. Richard trained as a clinical psychologist in Wellington, New Zealand where he worked in diverse settings including mental health, forensic psychology, private practice and neurology. His PhD examined the relationship between social support and stress among unemployed people and resulted in six publications in international journals. Richard taught psychology at Victoria University of Wellington, specializing in clinical neuropsychology, before joining the Rehabilitation Teaching and

Research Unit of the University of Otago in Wellington. Since then his teaching and research has focused on rehabilitation for neurological conditions. In 2007 he joined the staff of the Department of Palliative Care, Policy and Rehabilitation at King's College London where he was a Reader in Rehabilitation. In March 2012 he took up his current post. He is the author of 80 academic journal articles and six book chapters. Current research interests include psychometrics applied to neurological rehabilitation and palliative care, goal setting in rehabilitation and measuring community integration among people with complex disability.

William J. Taylor, PhD, MBChB, FAFRM, FRACP, Associate Professor in Rehabilitation Medicine, Rehabilitation Teaching and Research Unit, University of Otago Wellington and Consultant Rheumatologist and Rehabilitation Physician, Hutt Valley District Health Board, Wellington, New Zealand. Will trained in rheumatology and rehabilitation medicine, obtaining vocational registration in these areas in 1998. He continues to practise clinical medicine in Wellington, New Zealand. His PhD, partly based in Leeds United Kingdom, led to the widespread adoption of new classification criteria for the diagnosis of psoriatic arthritis. He now leads the Rehabilitation Teaching and Research Unit of the University of Otago Wellington, which is responsible for providing an interdisciplinary and distance-taught programme of studies in rehabilitation to postgraduate health professionals from diverse backgrounds. Will supervises research students and is actively involved in research in a variety of fields including vocational rehabilitation, goal setting, outcome measurement and clinical trial methodology (especially in gout and psoriatic arthritis). He works in collaboration with a number of local and overseas researchers including AUT University, OMERACT (Outcome Measures in Rheumatology Clinical Trials), GRAPPA (Group for Research and Assessment in Psoriasis and Psoriatic Arthritis) and the International Classification of Functioning, Disability and Health Research Centre. He has a particular interest in instrumentation, psychometrics and clinical epidemiology. A current research interest concerns response criteria following treatment for gout and classification criteria for gout. Will was a member of the New Zealand National Health Committee from 2007 to 2010, and is a member of the academic subcommittee of the ARFM (Australasian Faculty of Rehabilitation Medicine) and the continuing professional development subcommittee of the ARFM. He is the immediate past president of the New Zealand Rehabilitation Association.

About the contributors

Jo Adams, PhD, MSc, Dip COT, MBAOT, Senior Lecturer and Professional Lead for Occupational Therapy, Faculty of Health Sciences, University of Southampton United Kingdom. Jo is an occupational therapist who completed her clinical training at Cardiff. She has worked as an occupational therapist in the NHS, Social Services, higher education and within the voluntary sector in the United Kingdom, North America, Bangladesh and Uganda. Jo has a specialist interest in musculoskeletal rehabilitation and a particular focus on maximizing individuals' self-management skills and strategies across all groups of patients and clients. Her funded research projects involve close clinical collaboration with educationalists, rheumatologists, surgeons, engineers, nurses and therapists. Much of this collaborative work results in randomized controlled trials examining the clinical effectiveness of routine NHS clinical and educational interventions in rheumatology. Jo has for the past 16 years also been a keen and enthusiastic educator for undergraduate and postgraduate healthcare students striving to ensure that contemporary research and evidence-based practice is quickly embedded into healthcare education.

Claire Ballinger, PhD MSc Dip COT, Deputy Director/Senior Qualitative Health Research Fellow, National Institute for Health Research (NIHR) Research Design Service South Central, University of Southampton, United Kingdom. Claire qualified as an occupational therapist from Dorset House School of Occupational Therapy, Oxford, and worked with both older people, and people with learning disabilities for 8 years. She registered as a full-time student on the MSc in Rehabilitation Studies at the University of Southampton in 1989, and on graduating in 1991, took up her first academic post as a Lecturer in Rehabilitation at Southampton, evaluating disability equipment in the new Southampton Disability Equipment Assessment Centre. Claire joined the Southampton School of Occupational Therapy and Physiotherapy in 1994, and in 1996 was awarded a full time PhD research studentship by the Department of Health. After gaining her PhD in 2000, Claire became joint Head of Postgraduate Education in the School of Health Professions and Rehabilitation Sciences at Southampton before accepting a post as a Reader in Occupational Therapy at London South Bank University. She became a Professor of Occupational Therapy at Glasgow Caledonian University, before returning to Southampton to her current post in 2009.

Claire has a Visiting Chair at London South Bank University, and has recently reached the end of her term of office as Chair of the College of Occupational Therapists' Specialist Section – Older People. Her research interests include the design and evaluation of complex health interventions for older people, notably falls prevention, and she has particular expertise in qualitative research approaches, with a growing interest in randomized controlled trial design. Within the Research Design Service South Central, Claire has a strategic remit for patient and public involvement (PPI).

Szilvia Geyh, PhD, MPH, Dipl-Psych, Affiliated Teaching Fellow, Department of Health Sciences and Health Policy of the University of Lucerne, Switzerland. Szilvia is group leader at Swiss Paraplegic Research (SPF) and coordinates a research programme focusing on psychosocial and personal factors in spinal cord injury. Her teaching fellow position includes supporting PhD as well as master students. Szilvia holds a degree in psychology from the Catholic University of Eichstätt, a postgraduate master in public health and epidemiology as well as a PhD from the medical faculty of the Ludwig-Maximilian University (LMU) in Munich. Between 2001 and 2007 she worked as a research scientist in projects for the development and validation of the International Classification of Functioning, Disability, and Health (ICF) core sets for chronic health conditions at the Institute for Health and Rehabilitation Sciences of the LMU in collaboration with the World Health Organization (WHO). Her research interests circle around the comprehensive understanding of the lived experience of people with disabilities based on a biopsychosocial framework. Her work especially focuses on protective factors and psychosocial resources. She is also concerned with the conceptualization of the personal factors within WHO's ICF framework. Szilvia has a special interest in the problems of defining and measuring quality of life in people with disabilities, in person-centred rehabilitation and positive psychology. She has acted as a ICF trainer in national and international onsite, university and research workshops. She is specialized in the application of the ICF in neurological conditions, with a main focus on stroke and spinal cord injury. In addition, she has methodological expertise in Rasch analysis techniques for the evaluation and refinement of assessment instruments, and in conducting systematic literature reviews.

William Levack, PhD, MhealSc(Rehabilitation), BPhty, Associate Dean, Research and Postgraduate Studies for the University of Otago Wellington and Senior Lecturer in Rehabilitation for the Rehabilitation Teaching and Research Unit, Department of Medicine, University of Otago Wellington, New Zealand. William is a New Zealand registered physiotherapist who trained at the University of Otago. He began his clinical career working in New Zealand's public health system, primarily in services providing treatment and rehabilitation for aged-related neurological and respiratory conditions, before moving to help establish a new branch of a private residential rehabilitation service for people with acquired brain injury in the community. Afterwards, William returned to the public health system to work as the Physiotherapy Team Leader for Wellington Public Hospital, managing a team of 30 physiotherapists and support staff. In 2003, William was employed as a Lecturer at the University of Otago, teaching interdisciplinary, postgraduate courses in rehabilitation by distance, and in 2008 he completed his PhD. William's research interests include goal theory, patient engagement in rehabilitation and interprofessional rehabilitation processes. His current research projects includes work on the development of a clinical measure of loss and reconstruction of self-identity after traumatic brain injury, qualitative research into the barriers and facilitators of access to evidence-based rehabilitation, and the use of kinetic video games as a form of therapeutic exercise for people with chronic respiratory disease.

Julie Pryor, RN, RM, BA, GradCertRemoteHlthPrac, MN, PhD, FRCNA, Director of the Rehabilitation Nursing Research & Development Unit, Royal Rehabilitation Centre, Sydney, Australia. Julie is also an Associate Professor at Flinders University, where she contributes to Australia's only postgraduate multidisciplinary clinical rehabilitation programmes. She is a registered nurse with a passionate interest in rehabilitation. Since the mid-1980s Julie has held a variety of clinical, management, education and research positions in rehabilitation. Since the mid-1990s she has researched and published widely about rehabilitation, in particular nursing's role in rehabilitation, and provided consultancy advice to about 20 rehabilitation service providers across Australia and New Zealand. Julie's current areas of interest are making the person central to all the processes of clinical rehabilitation service delivery and the integration of clinical and community-based rehabilitation. She predominantly uses qualitative research methods and frequently works within a practice development framework.

Foreword
by Professor Gerold Stucki

Responding to a call by the World Health Assembly (2005) resolution on disability, including prevention, management and rehabilitation, the *World Report on Disability (WRD)* (World Health Organization (WHO), The World Bank, 2011) was launched at the United Nations headquarters in New York on 9 June 2011. By recognizing the *Convention on the Rights of Persons with Disabilities* (United Nations General Assembly, 2006) as its moral compass and the *International Classification of Functioning, Disability and Health (ICF)* (WHO, 2001) as its conceptual framework, the *WRD* provides rehabilitation practitioners and researchers worldwide with an influential global health policy reference.

The *WRD* defines rehabilitation as a set of measures that assist individuals 'who experience or are likely to experience disability to achieve and maintain optimal functioning in interaction with their environment' (2011, p. 308). This definition is based on the ICF framework and is consistent with the understanding of rehabilitation as a health strategy, complementing the preventive, curative and supportive health strategies (Meyer et al., 2011; Stucki et al., 2007a).

The *WRD* calls on countries 'to organize, strengthen, and extend comprehensive rehabilitation services and programmes' (2011, p. 95) and to strengthen rehabilitation research. A specific recommendation of the *WRD* is to develop 'models of service provision that encourage multidisciplinary and client-centred approaches' (2011, p. 123). This recommendation exactly represents the aim of *Interprofessional Rehabilitation*, edited by the three renowned experts in rehabilitation theory and practice: Sarah Dean, Richard Siegert and William Taylor.

Their book is the first work that provides rehabilitation practitioners and researchers with an in-depth discussion of the use of the ICF as a framework and as a language to structure the interprofessional rehabilitation process in interaction with the person in need of rehabilitation. The book comprehensively covers our current understanding of rehabilitation management, including an in-depth discussion of goal setting and a primer on the principles of outcome measurement. Most importantly, the book provides a chapter on 'The person in context', emphasizing and explaining what is referred to as 'in partnership between person and provider and in appreciation of the person's perception of his or her position in life' in the revised version of the ICF-based conceptual description of the rehabilitation strategy (Meyer et al., 2011, p. 767).

Wisely, the authors have decided to focus on core themes essential for a better understanding of interprofessional rehabilitation in light of the paradigm shift, from seeing disability either solely as the impact of a health condition or of the social environment, towards an integrative and universal model of functioning and disability. The sections on controversies, as well as the case studies, are a key strength of this book. They bring current debates – for example with respect to our understanding of activity and participation or with respect to the distinction of functioning versus quality of life – to the attention of the reader.

This book is proof that rehabilitation research, while still in its infancy, is well on its way towards becoming a truly scientific endeavour. Let me join the editors in their call to all readers to contribute to what, based on the ICF, can now be called 'human functioning and rehabilitation research' (Stucki et al., 2007b).

References

Meyer. T., Gutenbrunner, C., Bickenbach, J. E., Cieza, A., Melvin, J. and Stucki, G. (2011) Towards a conceptual description of rehabilitation as a health strategy. *Journal of Rehabilitation Medicine*, *43*, 765–769.

Stucki, G., Cieza, A. and Melvin, J. (2007a) The International Classification of Functioning, Disability and Health: a unifying model for the conceptual description of the rehabilitation strategy. *Journal of Rehabilitation Medicine*, *39*(4), 279–285.

Stucki, G., Reinhardt, J. D., Grimby, G. and Melvin, J. (2007b) Developing 'Human Functioning and Rehabilitation Research' from the comprehensive perspective. *Journal of Rehabilitation Medicine*, *39*(9), 665–671.

United Nations General Assembly. (2006) *Convention on the Rights of Persons with Disabilities. Resolution 61/106*. New York: United Nations

World Health Assembly. (2005) *Disability, including Prevention, Management and Rehabilitation. Resolution 58.23*. Geneva: World Health Assembly.

World Health Organization. (2001) *International Classification of Functioning, Disability and Health*. Geneva: WHO.

World Health Organization, The World Bank. (2011) *World Report on Disability*. Geneva: WHO.

Gerold Stucki, MD, MS
Professor and Chair, Department of Health Sciences and Health Policy,
University of Lucerne, Lucerne, Switzerland,
Director, Swiss Paraplegic Research and ICF Research Branch
of the WHO FIC CC in Germany (at DIMDI), Nottwil, Switzerland

Preface

We wrote this book with the aim of providing a concise and readable introduction to the principles and practice of an interprofessional approach to rehabilitation that places the patient or client in their specific personal context. It is our belief that effective rehabilitation is best conducted by well-integrated teams of specialists working in an interdisciplinary way with the client or patient actively involved in all stages of the process. It is our hope that we will convince most of the readers of this book to share in this belief. However, beliefs are just that – beliefs – and they not to be confused with facts. So we would like to preface this book by giving some explanation for our own belief in the notion that rehabilitation is, or should be, both interprofessional and person centred.

We base this belief on three different strands of evidence. The first is our own subjective personal experiences of working as health professionals in various rehabilitation settings. The second line of evidence is also rather subjective in nature although it does at least involve a much larger sample size. It is the consensus wisdom, gleaned from several hundred experienced health professionals working in rehabilitation, who have completed and contributed to the courses in rehabilitation that we teach. The third source of evidence for our belief in the interprofessional, person-centred approach to rehabilitation is more objective and so has more scientific credibility. It stems from the growing body of published research on rehabilitation and its many facets. Much of this research will be summarized, analysed, debated and critiqued in the following pages as we outline our own perspective on rehabilitation. In reading this new text *Interprofessional Rehabilitation: A patient centred-approach* we would like to invite you, the reader, to adopt a similar three-pronged strategy in accepting or rejecting our belief in the person-centred and interprofessional nature of rehabilitation.

In other words we ask that you read the book and examine its message in the light of three separate kinds of evidence: (1) your own day-to-day clinical experience, (2) the opinions of workmates and colleagues from your own and allied disciplines, and (3) the scientific evidence. In many respects the purpose of this book is to provide the third component i.e. the scientific or research evidence. What the book cannot provide is the more 'subjective' evidence for a belief in a person-centred, interprofessional approach to rehabilitation. As we noted above, this kind of evidence is best found through your own thinking and reflection about your clinical practice and also through discussions and debates with colleagues. We hope that this book offers some challenges to your ways of thinking and provides a sound introduction to person-centred interprofessional rehabilitation based upon a firm scientific evidence base. We also hope that you will supplement this evidence by testing most of what you read against your own daily experience in the clinic and through discussions with your colleagues and patients. In particular we welcome your feedback, suggestions, comments, criticism, praise, insights and anecdotes about how you found this book helpful or otherwise in your workplace.

Sarah G. Dean, Richard J. Siegert and William J. Taylor

Acknowledgements

We gratefully acknowledge current and previous staff of the Rehabilitation Teaching and Research Unit, University of Otago, Wellington in New Zealand, who have made significant contributions to the ideas expressed in this book. In particular, we would like to acknowledge the seminal contribution of Professor Kath McPherson and Dr Harry McNaughton for their vision of interprofessional education in rehabilitation, as well as Dr Jean Hay-Smith, Ms Ginny Hickman, Dr William Levack, Dr Sue Lord, Ms Anne Sinnott and Professor Mark Weatherall for their contribution in identifying and developing the five core themes promoted in this book.

We also acknowledge and thank Dr Anna Sansom for her assistance with preparing the manuscript.

Dr Sarah Dean's time was partially supported by the National Institute for Health Research (NIHR) UK. However, the views expressed are those of the author and not necessarily those of the NIHR or the UK Department of Health.

Financial support for Professor Richard Siegert's time in the preparation of the manuscript was provided by the Dunhill Medical Trust and the Luff Foundation.

Chapter 1

Introduction

Richard J. Siegert,[1] *William J. Taylor*[2]
and Sarah G. Dean[3]

[1]*Professor of Psychology and Rehabilitation, School of Rehabilitation and Occupation Studies and School of Public Health and Psychosocial Studies, AUT University, Auckland, New Zealand;* [2]*Associate Professor in Rehabilitation Medicine, Rehabilitation Teaching and Research Unit, University of Otago Wellington and Consultant Rheumatologist and Rehabilitation Physician, Hutt Valley District Health Board, Wellington, New Zealand;* [3]*Senior Lecturer in Health Services Research, University of Exeter Medical School, United Kingdom*

1.1   What is rehabilitation?

As academics we are in the habit of defining any important terms that we use in our teaching or research publications and this is a practice that we expect from our students in their assignments. So it is hard to avoid starting a textbook on rehabilitation without defining precisely what we mean by this word. But at the same time a part of us already knows that we are doomed to fail in this rather ambitious task. Why this sense of pessimism?

It may be that it stems from our having sat through too many lengthy and heated discussions at learned conferences about how best to define rehabilitation. It is actually hard to find the right words to capture all the meanings that rehabilitation has for different people. It is especially hard to do this in a few pithy sentences since we all have different perspectives on rehabilitation depending on whether we are a health professional, a client or patient, a caregiver or relative of a patient, or a health manager with budgetary responsibility.

Or it might come from the knowledge that the field subsumes such a wide range of diseases and health conditions across the lifespan and such a growing range of methods for assessing and intervening in these conditions. So the physiotherapist who works with a 7-year-old boy with cerebral palsy to improve his gait is engaging in rehabilitation. Similarly the nurse who specializes in continence management in adults with multiple sclerosis is engaged in rehabilitation. But what about the physiotherapist

Interprofessional Rehabilitation: A Person-Centred Approach, First Edition.
Edited by Sarah G. Dean, Richard J. Siegert and William J. Taylor.
© 2012 John Wiley & Sons, Ltd. Published 2012 by John Wiley & Sons, Ltd.

who works with an elderly man in the end stage of heart failure to maximize his strength, mobility and quality of life? Is this rehabilitation or palliative care?

Notwithstanding these concerns we shall begin this text on rehabilitation with a fairly searching consideration – what exactly is rehabilitation. To do this we will first clarify what rehabilitation is not – or at least what we the authors do not include as rehabilitation for the purposes of this book. Then we will consider a number of definitions that other authors have offered and attempt to tease out some of the key ideas that they share and also the problematic issues in arriving at a consensus definition of rehabilitation. Next, we will introduce the five core concepts that lie at the heart of this book. These core concepts will, to a large extent, define what we understand by the term rehabilitation. However, we will not conclude this chapter by selecting or proposing a single, 'best' definition of rehabilitation. Rather, we prefer to let all these definitions and concepts, ideas and opinions, percolate for a time while we examine our core themes in depth. Having completed that journey we will then ask you, in Chapter 7, to revisit the issue of how we might best define rehabilitation.

1.2   Setting boundaries – or what we don't mean by rehabilitation

The word 'rehabilitation' has become a buzzword in the early 21st century. Wherever you look there is somebody using the word rehabilitation. But depending on who is talking or writing, who is being rehabilitated and the context in which they are using it, the meaning can vary considerably. Hardly a day goes by without us reading in the tabloid press about the latest film star or pop singer to go into 'rehab'. Our daily papers also feature heated arguments in the Letters to the Editor section about the merits of spending taxes on trying to 'rehabilitate' hardened criminals – or whether we should simply be locking them away for longer sentences. Not so long ago dissident politicians in some communist countries occasionally disappeared from public life only to reappear some years later having been politically 'rehabilitated'. A famous example of this was Deng Xiaoping who fell from grace during the Cultural Revolution but was later 'rehabilitated' and eventually became the leader of the People's Republic of China. In searching electronic databases for our own research, using rehabilitation as keyword, we discovered that the term is also commonly used for the process of restoring land that has been ravaged by mining.

Interestingly, although none of these uses of the word have any great relevance for our text, they do all convey the sense of someone or something that has in some way become damaged or corrupted and then, through some prolonged process, has been restored to an acceptable or desirable state of existence.

However, we wish to be quite clear in this book, that in using the term rehabilitation, we are not referring to interventions for substance misuse problems, criminal offending, (perceived) political misdemeanours or natural environments devastated by human technology. In general we will use the term only for referring to ways of working with people who have some type of disability resulting from a congenital, traumatic or chronic health condition. Some examples of these conditions are amputations, cerebral palsy, chronic obstructive pulmonary disease, lower back pain, multiple sclerosis, myocardial infarction, Parkinson's disease, spinal cord injury, stroke, schizophrenia and traumatic brain injury. However, this is starting to sound like a definition of rehabilitation, so it might be a good point to consider some of the ways in which other people have already defined the concept.

1.3   Some definitions of rehabilitation

Chambers Twentieth Century Dictionary gives the following definition of rehabilitate 'to reinstate, restore to former privileges, rights, rank etc,: to clear the charter of: to bring back into good condition, working order, prosperity: to make fit, after disablement or illness, for earning a living or playing a part in the world' (Macdonald, 1974, p. 1138)

The word rehabilitation comes from the Latin root 'habil' meaning to enable. Rehabilitation therefore means to 're-enable' or 'restore' and it is this sense of the word that is captured above in the diverse meanings attributed to it. However, our concern is primarily with the use of the word within healthcare and related settings. Rehabilitation is a relatively new term and specialty within healthcare (Gritzer and Arluke, 1985). One of the earlier definitions of rehabilitation within the healthcare realm is Jefferson's (1941) statement that rehabilitation should be: '...the planned attempt under skilled direction by the use of all available measures to restore or improve the health, usefulness and happiness of those who have suffered injury or are recovering from disease. Its further object is to return them to the service of the community in the shortest time' (Jefferson, 1941).

Notwithstanding its age, this statement of Jefferson's captures a number of key ideas that are integral to the aims and purposes of contemporary rehabilitation practitioners. There is the implication that rehabilitation is a complex process demanding a high level of professional skill and a holistic view of the individual. It is also clear from this definition that rehabilitation is not just about restoring or improving the person's physical health – their happiness is also vitally important. Even more contemporary is the assertion that rehabilitation enables the individual, not merely to feed and clothe themselves, but to participate as a citizen who makes an important contribution to their community.

Some 40 years after Jefferson, the World Health Organization (WHO), advanced the following definition: 'Rehabilitation is a problem-solving and educational process aimed at reducing the disability and handicap experienced by someone as a result of disease, always within the limitations imposed by available resources and the underlying disease' (cited in Wade, 1992, p. 11).

This definition highlights a shift in thinking about rehabilitation as largely a medical concern, to a broader concern with the person's biological, psychological and social functioning i.e. the biopsychosocial model. Thus, rehabilitation is not simply a medical concern but requires the person to learn new skills and ways of coping with their changed circumstances. The following definition from Barnes and Ward (2000, p. 4) is very similar in emphasizing rehabilitation as an educational or learning process that has physical, psychological and social dimensions: 'Rehabilitation can thus be defined as an active and dynamic process by which a disabled person is helped to acquire knowledge and skills in order to maximize physical, psychological, and social function. It is a process that maximizes functional ability and minimizes disability and handicap'.

The final definition that we wish to consider here comes from Sinclair and Dickinson (1998, p. 1): 'a process aiming to restore personal autonomy in those aspects of daily living considered most relevant by patients, service users and their family carers'. This concise statement emphasizes two key elements of modern rehabilitation practice that will also be emphasized in this book. First, is the notion that the most important goals in the rehabilitation process are those that matter most to the client or patient and only they can identify these goals. The second is the awareness that the patient's family, relatives, caregivers, friends etc. are important participants in a good rehabilitation programme.

1.4   Some other issues in defining rehabilitation

Before introducing the five core themes of this book there are a couple of additional issues in defining rehabilitation that we need to consider. The first is the difference between *therapy* and *rehabilitation*. The second concerns a particularly strong challenge to traditional notions of rehabilitation and disability that arose in the 1970s.

Therapy versus rehabilitation

A major part of any programme of rehabilitation consists of the different kinds of therapies involved. These typically include occupational therapy, physiotherapy, and speech and language therapy (DeJong et al., 2005). These 'core therapies' may be supplemented with interventions offered by podiatrists, psychologists, social workers, family therapists, sport and exercise therapists, and experts in the use of assistive technologies. However, 'doing' therapy is not the same thing as 'doing' rehabilitation and rehabilitation is not just a synonym for therapies. Even worse is the assumption that after a spell in the neurosurgical, geriatric or orthopaedic ward, a patient enters 'rehabilitation' prior to discharge into the community.

The point at issue here is simply that rehabilitation means more than just physical therapy or spending two weeks in a ward with that name. It is actually about a comprehensive approach to working with the person and their family. This kind of approach can occur in an acute setting, a designated rehabilitation ward and also in the community until long after discharge from hospital. Moreover, some therapists practice therapy without a rehabilitation approach whereas some non-therapists (e.g. family, friends, community nurses, general practitioners) play an active role in the rehabilitation process. In other words, although the various therapies are essential to rehabilitation, they are still only components of a broader and more complex process.

Disabling societies

Perhaps the strongest challenge yet to traditional medical understanding of how to best define rehabilitation has come from disability rights activists and academics in the field of disability studies (Braddock and Parish, 2001; Fougeyrollas and Beauregard, 2001). After the growth and influence of the civil rights movement in the USA in the1960s, the flourishing of the women's movement in many countries, and an increasing awareness of the rights of psychiatric patients, the1970s were a period of rapid growth in political activism among disabled people. The 1970s also saw the emergence of the social model of disability (Braddock and Parish, 2001). There are different perspectives on what exactly the social model of disability is and its implications but the following quotation from David Pfeiffer captures its essence nicely: 'Disability is not a medical nor a health question. It is a policy or political issue. A disability comes not from the existence of an impairment, but from the reality of building codes, educational practices, stereotypes, prejudicial public officials (judges, administrators, direct care workers), ignorance, and oppression which results in some people facing discrimination while others benefit from those acts of discrimination' (Pfeiffer, 1999, p. 106).

In this passage Pfeiffer is arguing that disablement is not merely the natural consequence of some biological defect within the individual but rather a form of discrimination or oppression that society inflicts upon those people who are perceived or labelled as physically or mentally impaired. Hence disability (and presumably rehabilitation too) is a political issue rather than just a medical or health issue. So, from this perspective, disability is more a reflection of how much a society values differences among people and allocates its resources to ensure that all people have the opportunity to participate fully in society. For example, disability is partly a product of architecture and buildings that for centuries were designed without even considering their accessibility for disabled people. Or to take another example, disability is a result of a competitive job market that actively or subtly discriminates against people with disabilities.

The arguments for and against a social model of disability are well beyond the scope of the present text (readers wishing to learn more about the social model of disability and different perspectives on it would do well to consult recent issues of the journal *Disability and Society* published by Taylor and Francis). However, the social model of disability has had a substantial and lasting impact on contemporary perspectives on rehabilitation. Evidence of this impact can be seen in the World Health Organization's (WHO) system for the classification of the 'consequences of disease' and its evolution since 1980. One of the most noticeable changes in the evolution from the International Classification of Impairment, Disease and Handicap (ICIDH) through the ICIDH-2 to the current International Classification of Functioning (ICF) (WHO, 2001) is the greater emphasis that is given to the role of environmental factors (social and physical) in contributing to the process of disablement. Concomitant with this shift has been a transition from a largely biomedical or disease model to a biopsy-chosocial approach. Interestingly, the introduction to the ICF describes both the medical and the social models of disability and functioning and notes that the 'ICF is based on an integration of these two opposing models' (WHO, 2001, p. 20). We propose that the ICF provides a framework for rehabilitation, and is therefore the first core theme for this book (see Chapter 2).

The impact of the social model of disability is also reflected in the present book – most notably in Chapter 6, which is about the person in context. However, this book is written by academic health professionals, who have all worked in a range of reha-bilitation settings, and so it will also reflect many aspects of the traditional medical model. There are risks involved in asserting that disability is purely a social construc-tion and not a medical issue. One of these risks is that we ignore the reality that many disabled people are high frequency users of the health system. Their lives bring them into all too regular contact with health professionals. Consequently, in this book we adopt a perspective akin to that advocated by the ICF in which the aim is to bridge these two opposing viewpoints and to integrate biological, psychological and social elements of rehabilitation.

1.5   The core themes

Having set the scene we now introduce the five core themes that make up the content of Chapters 2 to 6 of this book. As we have mentioned, the first theme concerns the ICF, how this can be used as a framework for rehabilitation and act as a model and classification system. This chapter has been written by William Taylor, a rheumatolo-gist who has worked on the use of the ICF for people with psoriatic arthritis, and by Szilvia Geyh, a psychologist who has worked for the ICF Research Branch in co-operation with the WHO Collaborating Centre for the Family of International Classifications in Germany (at DIMDI – the German Institute of Medical Documentation and Information). William and Szilvia's chapter describes the ICF, its development and terminology, and how it can be used for assessment and interven-tion evaluation. They go on to discuss the limitations and controversies about the ICF and its future development. The next theme concerns interprofessional rehabilitation and this chapter (Chapter 3) has been written by two allied health professionals who have worked clinically in rehabilitation settings (occupational therapy and physio-therapy) but who have also been lecturers involved with delivering interprofessional education. Claire Ballinger and Sarah Dean discuss teamwork and the roles and make-up of successful rehabilitation teams including service users.

After this, Chapter 4 goes on to describe the processes by which these teams engage in doing rehabilitation. William Levack, a physiotherapist, takes the lead on this chapter, and in particular provides a detailed account of one of the key processes in rehabilitation: goal setting. By the end of Chapter 4 we hope to have made it clear that the rehabilitation processes theme also includes the process of evaluating practice.

Outcome evaluation is therefore the next core theme and this is covered in much more detail in Chapter 5 by Richard Siegert, an expert in the development and evaluation of rehabilitation outcome measures, and by Jo Adams, an occupational therapist with expertise in the development, application and research of outcome measures for people with hand impairments. Our final core theme, the person in context, is placed last in our list of themes, not because it is the least important but rather because it is the ultimate focus of all our themes. The earlier chapters all touch on how the patient, client or service user is the focus of rehabilitation and in Chapter 6 Julie Pryor, nurse and director of a Nursing Rehabilitation Research and Development Unit in Australia, leads the discussion on how to place the person in their context and the importance of this for successful and meaningful rehabilitation to take place.

1.6   A word about terminology

Throughout the book we have asked our authors to consider the terminology they are using and to provide definitions as appropriate. However, in many instances there are several terms that can be used interchangeably, for example patient, client, or person can all be used to prefix 'centred care'. Rather than attempt to be popular or to be prescriptive in our terminology, we will use whichever word provides the best fit for the sentence in question. For example, the term 'patient-centred care' is often used in this book because it clearly identifies the person in question, differentiating them from say, relatives or carers.

1.7   Summary

The final chapter of this book (Chapter 7) revisits the key messages of our five core themes; identifies the limitations in current thinking and practice and suggests some of the likely developments for the future of rehabilitation. We hope that you will enjoy this book; it is not profession or discipline specific but does cover a range of examples from differing conditions, rehabilitation approaches and types of research. Thus, we believe there is something here for everyone involved in interprofessional rehabilitation.

References

Barnes, M. P. and Ward, A. B. (2000). *Textbook of Rehabilitation Medicine*. Oxford: Oxford University Press.

Braddock, D. L. and Parish, S. L. (2001). An institutional history of disability. In: G. L. Albrecht, K. D. Seelman and M. Bury. *Handbook of Disability Studies*. Thousand Oaks, CA: Sage Publications.

DeJong, G., Horn, S. D., Conway, B., Nichols, D. and Healton, E. B. (2005). Opening the black box of poststroke rehabilitation: stroke rehabilitation patients, processes, and outcomes. *Archives of Physical Medicine and Rehabilitation*, 86(Supplement 1), 1–7.

Fougeyrollas, P. and Beauregard, L. (2001). An interactive person-environment social creation. In: G. L. Albrecht, K. D. Seelman and M. Bury. *Handbook of Disability Studies*. Thousand Oaks, CA: Sage Publications.

Gritzer, G. and Arluke, A. (1985). *The Making of Rehabilitation: A Political Economy of Medical Specialization 1890–1980*. Berkeley, CA: University of California Press.

Jefferson, G. (1941). Discussion on rehabilitation after injuries to the central nervous system. *Proceedings of the Royal Society of Medicine*, *35*, 295–299.

Macdonald, A. M. (1974). *Chambers Twentieth Century Dictionary*. Edinburgh: W & R Chambers.

Pfeiffer, D. (1999). The categorization and control of people with disabilities. *Disability and Rehabilitation*, *21*(3), 106–107.

Sinclair, A. and Dickinson, E. (1998). *Effective Practice in Rehabilitation*. London: King's Fund Publishing.

Wade, D. T. (1992). *Measurement in Neurological Rehabilitation*. Oxford: Oxford University Press.

World Health Organization. (2001). *International Classification of Functioning, Disability and Health: ICF*. Geneva: World Health Organization.

Chapter 2

A rehabilitation framework: the International Classification of Functioning, Disability and Health

William J. Taylor[1] and Szilvia Geyh[2,3]

[1]*Associate Professor in Rehabilitation Medicine, Rehabilitation Teaching and Research Unit, University of Otago Wellington and Consultant Rheumatologist and Rehabilitation Physician, Hutt Valley District Health Board, Wellington, New Zealand;* [2]*Affiliated Teaching Fellow, Department of Health Sciences and Health Policy of the University of Lucerne, Switzerland;* [3]*Group Leader at Swiss Paraplegic Research, Nottwil, Switzerland*

2.1 There is a need for a common language of functioning

It is hard to overestimate the importance of good communication between rehabilitation health professionals from different disciplines involved in the care of the same client. The different 'life worlds' of people from diverse backgrounds can lead to talking past each other, miscommunication or misunderstanding. Imagine the following conversation at a weekly inpatient rehabilitation team meeting.

DOCTOR: When is Mr Brown likely to be ready to be discharged? He is *walking well* now and does not seem especially *disabled*.

PHYSIOTHERAPIST: Yes but he is still *getting stronger* and will be able to walk better if he receives more therapy. His *ankle dorsiflexors are still not functioning very well* at all.

NURSE: He is totally *independent with self-cares*.

DOCTOR: Well then we could plan to discharge tomorrow then.

OCCUPATIONAL THERAPIST: He *manages fine in the ward* but he has stairs at home and I don't know how well he will *cope with that environment*.

SOCIAL WORKER: He wants to be home as quickly as possible and back at work because financially things are tight for his family. He is *actually doing some work* in hospital since most of it is computer-based.

PHYSIOTHERAPIST: Well, what are the priorities – shouldn't we be getting him as *functional as possible*? Isn't that our job?

In this exchange, a number of words relating to the concept of 'functioning' are in italic. There appears to be different concepts about what this means among the different health professionals, yet many would probably agree with the physiotherapist's belief that the primary task of rehabilitation is to maximize the person's level of 'functioning'. A key issue then, in order for rehabilitation teams to work productively together, is to agree upon what is meant by this important term. As we see in this hypothetical exchange, 'functioning' can refer to how well a person walks, the strength of a particular muscle, ability to perform a task within one environment compared with a different environment, self-care activities or actual performance of productive work.

The doctor and nurse seem to believe that accomplishment of a particular task (such as walking or self-care activities) renders the person non-disabled, irrespective of how difficult or how 'well' that task is managed. Furthermore, they ignore the possibility that a person can function quite well in one environment but not in another. Contextual factors are clearly more important than they realize. The occupational therapist is much more aware of the more nuanced notion of disability in which the environment can render the person disabled rather than the intrinsic abilities of the person. In such situations, improving a person's function may have nothing to do with more therapy, but rather requires a change to the environment, such as building a ramp rather than steps. Functioning must therefore be seen as an interaction between the person and their context. One other important consideration of 'context', which was not raised by the team discussion, is the context of the person himself. That is, what attributes (not directly related to the issue at hand) does the client bring. This can involve his age, co-morbidities and personality traits among a range of possibilities. This context too is very important in determining the actual functioning of the person.

The social worker introduces two additional concepts. The first concerns a distinction between more basic activities such as walking and those that are more societal in orientation – fulfilling a role such as paid work or being part of a family. Accomplishing such a role may often have little relation to more basic activities, and therefore cannot be seen as hierarchical. In this example, it is simply not necessary for the person to be able to walk well in order for him to perform his paid work. Of course, in other kinds of work, walking will be a pre-requisite. But the relationship between specific disturbances of basic activities (which we might consider as those occurring at the level of the whole organism), and other kinds of activities such as work (which we might consider at the level of organism within his/her social world) cannot be assumed and needs to be evaluated carefully as part of good rehabilitation practice for each client. The second concept that the social worker introduces is the notion of 'actual performance' perhaps, as if this was a more impressive observation than 'is capable of'. Certainly, the two concepts are distinct. Direct observation of performance is possible but determining capacity is rather more judgemental and involves making a prediction rather than describing what is observed. Whether observation of performance is better than prediction of capacity is unclear and almost certainly depends upon what the evaluation is used for – is it fit for purpose? Often a determination of performance is not possible, since the particular activity occurs very infrequently or is potentially dangerous. For example, how could the team respond to Mr Browns's request for some guidance as to whether he can engage in his hobby of skydiving?

Returning to the physiotherapist again, the common use of the term 'function' that is synonymous with 'operate' means that how well or poorly parts of the organism are working also comes under the umbrella of 'function'. Again, the relationship between the operation of parts of the organism and the whole of the organism are not necessarily hierarchical or linear. Walking is possible without all components of the walking mechanism working normally (or at all). Entire loss of a lower limb does not preclude walking. It is often critically important for therapists to consider carefully the primary targets of their treatment and to constantly re-evaluate the relevance of that target in relation to the overall rehabilitation plan.

It is clearly necessary, therefore, to organize these different concepts of 'functioning' into a schema that all disciplines can understand and use. We might consider this a common language of functioning where each term is precisely defined and meaningful across the different discipline-specific languages. For example, when occupational therapists talk about the 'Model of Human Occupation' (Kielhofner, 2008), can the language be translated into the same terms that psychologists would use when discussing 'cognitive–behavioural therapy'?

From the perspective of populations, healthcare systems and payers such a language is also important. For example, a means of how to classify, categorize and enumerate all the ways people are affected by health conditions is necessary in order to properly understand the health and functioning of a population. A descriptive language that contains all the manifestations of health and disease would be complementary to a descriptive system of pathological diagnoses contained within the International Classification of Disease (ICD) (WHO, 1992).

This chapter discusses such a language. The International Classification of Functioning, Disability and Health (ICF) introduced by the World Health Organization (WHO) in 2001 was a landmark achievement towards comprehensively understanding and describing 'functioning' (Ustun et al., 2003). With this language, it is now possible for different disciplines to understand what each other does and begin to form rational commonalities across discipline-specific models of thinking. Furthermore, an acceptable language of functioning enables a more scientific discourse to determine the nature of functioning in its totality and in its component parts. The better way of describing functioning that the ICF provides can permit an investigation into the connections between its component parts, the determinants of functioning and the effectiveness of interventions that might improve functioning. It may not be overstating the case to say that the ICF is a central pillar of rehabilitation theory and practice.

This chapter will describe the origin of the ICF, describe the ICF in more detail, explain the core set and other approaches to making the ICF more usable, and how the ICF relates to measurement of functioning and health status. We will discuss some difficulties with the ICF – in particular how it relates to quality of life (QoL) – and the distinctions between some components of the ICF. And finally we consider some possible developments for the future of the ICF.

2.2   The ICF is both a model and a classification system

Introduction

The endorsement of the ICF (WHO, 2001) by the World Health Assembly in May 2001 was a milestone that gave important impetus to health services provision and research, especially to the field of rehabilitation (Stucki et al., 2002). Traditionally, functioning and disability have been considered as the *result* or *consequence*, caused and fully determined by disease or injury. This idea is expressed by the so-called medical or bio-medical model (Boorse, 1975, 1977). However, functioning and disability are more complex than this. In reality it is apparent that the disease or injury (described by a diagnosis) is not sufficient to determine the functioning and disability of individuals (WHO, 2002). Two people with the same diagnosis can often have different levels of functioning and disability, whereas a similar pattern of functioning and disability may result from different aetiologies. For example, a rupture of the anterior cruciate ligament will lead to different consequences for a 28-year-old professional soccer player compared with a 64-year-old grandmother living on the fourth floor of a building without an elevator. A diagnosis alone does not sufficiently explain, for example, length of hospital stay, the required amount of nursing care or therapy applications. A diagnosis of a pathological process does not describe an individual person's level of persistent disability, his or her ability to return to work, or the potential for community reintegration.

Healthcare planning, management, evaluation and funding, in the clinical, institutional or policy context, needs more information beyond the diagnosis. The ICF has been developed to complement the diagnostic information. A standardized systematic terminology has been available for diseases for over a hundred years, namely the most recent version of the International Classification of Diseases (ICD-10, WHO, 1992). In contrast, the ICF as a globally agreed common language and a framework for the description of the components of health, functioning and disability was first published in 2001. Whereas detailed statistics on prevalence, incidence and mortality of diseases are available, much less is known about the health states of people with chronic conditions and the survivors of acute events, like stroke or spinal cord injury.

The ICF is both a basic model for the comprehensive understanding of health and health-related states and the classification that implements the model and provides a multipurpose, systematic and universal language to describe a wide range of health-related phenomena.

The ICF as a model

The ICF is based upon a comprehensive *biopsychosocial model*, which integrates different perspectives of health into one unified and coherent view. What does this mean? The model is comprehensive as it includes various dimensions, i.e. it considers disability not only from a physical, but also from an individual and societal perspective, and importantly includes the environmental and personal context of the

Table 2.1 The International Classification of Functioning, Disability and Health (ICF) components and their definitions.

Parts	Components	Definition
Health condition	Health condition	disease (acute or chronic), disorder, injury or trauma
Functioning and disability	Body functions	are the physiological functions of body systems
	Body structures	are anatomical parts of the body such as organs, limbs and their components
	Impairments	are problems in body function or structure such as a significant deviation or loss
	Activity	is the execution of a task or action by an individual
	Activity limitations	are difficulties an individual may have in executing activities
	Participation	is involvement in life situation
	Participation restrictions	are problems an individual may experience in involvement in life situations
Contextual factors	Environmental factors	make up the physical, social and attitudinal environment in which people live and conduct their lives
	Personal factors	are the particular background of an individual's life and living, and comprise features of the individual that are not part of a health condition or health states

individual. It is integrative as it combines biomedical, psychological as well as social views of disability.

Components of the ICF model

The biopsychosocial model consists of three parts: (1) the health condition, (2) functioning with its three main components, and (3) the two contextual factors. The model comprises six building blocks, which address the six components of health: the health condition, body functions and structures, activity, participation, environmental factors and personal factors. These components taken together provide a full picture of functioning, disability and health. The ICF presents definitions for all of these components, which are shown in Table 2.1.

Health condition refers to any kind of disorder or disease, but also to further phenomena, e.g. trauma, congenital anomalies, genetic predispositions or ageing. Functioning embraces three dimensions that refer to different perspectives, namely, the perspective of the human body, of the whole individual and of society. The first dimension, representing the level of the body, includes body functions and body structures. Body functions are the physiological functions of body systems, also including mental functions. Body structures are the anatomical parts of the body. Activity represents the individual perspective of functioning. Activity is described as the execution of a task or action by an individual as an independent subject. Participation is the involvement of the individual in life situations. It represents the societal perspective of functioning.

The contextual factors include the environmental factors and the personal factors. Environmental factors refer to the physical, social and attitudinal environment that form the context of an individual's life and, as such, have an impact on the person's functioning. Personal factors are contextual factors that make up the particular background of an individual's life and living, but are not part of the health condition or health states. For example, age, gender, social status, life experiences, personality, etc.

The central concepts of the biopsychosocial model are functioning and disability. Functioning is an umbrella term for intact body functions and structures, activities and participation. Functioning denotes the positive or neutral outcome of the bidirectional complex interaction between an individual's health condition and his or her context. The complementary term disability is an umbrella term to denote impairments of body functions and structures, activity limitations or participation restrictions, which are the negative aspects of the named interaction.

The current understanding of the interactions of the components of functioning, disability and health within the biopsychosocial approach is depicted in Figure 2.1. It is important to note that the components of the ICF model relate to each other in a complex bidirectional way, as opposed to a linear–causal type of relationship.

Case study

Lucy is a 38-year-old woman who has had rheumatoid arthritis. She has severe deformities of her hands and feet, and cannot grip strongly or walk far. She is the chief executive officer of a multinational company and is married with two primary-school age children. Her company is supportive of flexible working practices. She describes herself as determined and a 'big-picture person'.

Considering the ICF model and the information from this brief description, the 'functioning' and other components of the model for Lucy would be considered in the following terms:

- Health condition: rheumatoid arthritis
- Body structures and functions : pain, deformity and impaired movement of several joints
- Activity limitations: gripping difficulties, walking long distances
- Participation restrictions: none
- Environmental factors: supportive employer
- Personal factors: determined and well-balanced personality

The ICF as a classification

The integrative biopsychosocial framework of the ICF is implemented in the according classification. The classification is the flesh to the skeleton of the model framework. The common *idea* of the model is represented by the standardized *language* or terminology of the classification.

The ICF as a classification is a listing of categories that fully describes the various aspects of functioning and the environment, organized within components. The

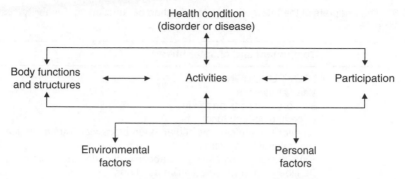

Figure 2.1 The biopsychosocial model of functioning, disability and health. (With permission from the World Health Organization see http://www.who.int/classifications/icf/en/)

Table 2.2 The nested structure of the International Classification of Functioning, Disability and Health (ICF).

Code	Category	Level
b	*Body functions*	
b1	*Mental functions*	(first/chapter level)
b114	*Orientation functions*	(second level)
b1142	*Orientation to person*	(third level)
b11420	*Orientation to self*	(fourth level)
b11421	*Orientation to others*	(fourth level)

categories are structured in a hierarchically nested way. Each component consists of chapters (categories at the first level), each chapter consists of second-level categories, and in turn they are made up of categories at the third and fourth levels. The ICF provides categories for the different kinds of body functions, a list of body structures, a joint list of activities and participations, and a list of environmental factors. An example to illustrate the nested structure of the ICF is presented in Table 2.2.

Table 2.3 shows the available chapters of the ICF. The 30 chapters include overall 1424 categories at the second, third and fourth levels. The categories are accompanied by definitions, examples, inclusion and exclusion criteria. The total list can be viewed using the Manual available from the WHO or by using the online ICF browser (http://apps.who.int/classifications/icfbrowser/).

Personal factors are not yet implemented as a part of the classification. Moreover, health conditions are not classified by the ICF, but are classified by another member of the WHO family of international classifications, the ICD-10 (WHO, 1992).

The ICF states that the description of the functioning of a person is not complete without adding to the ICF categories the so called 'qualifiers'. The qualifiers denote the *extent* of impairments, limitations and restrictions. They quantify the level of functioning and health or the severity of the problem in the different ICF categories. The WHO proposes that all categories of the classification are to be quantified using the same generic scale ranging from 0 (no problem) to 4 (complete problem). In the

Table 2.3   The chapters of the International Classification of Functioning, Disability and Health (ICF).

Code	Component and chapter titles
b	BODY FUNCTIONS
b1	Mental functions
b2	Sensory functions and pain
b3	Voice and speech functions
b4	Functions of the cardiovascular, haematological, immunological and respiratory systems
b5	Functions of the digestive, metabolic and endocrine systems
b6	Genitourinary and reproductive functions
b7	Neuromusculoskeletal and movement-related functions
b8	Functions of the skin and related structures
s	BODY STRUCTURES
s1	Structures of the nervous system
s2	The eye, ear and related structures
s3	Structures involved in voice and speech
s4	Structures of the cardiovascular, immunological and respiratory systems
s5	Structures related to the digestive, metabolic and endocrine systems
s6	Structures related to the genitourinary and reproductive systems
s7	Structures related to movement
s8	Skin and related structures
d	ACTIVITY AND PARTICIPATION
d1	Learning and applying knowledge
d2	General tasks and demands
d3	Communication
d4	Mobility
d5	Self-care
d6	Domestic life
d7	Interpersonal interactions and relationships
d8	Major life areas
d9	Community, social and civic life
e	ENVIRONMENTAL FACTORS
e1	Products and technology
e2	Natural environment and human-made changes to environment
e3	Support and relationships
e4	Attitudes
e5	Services, systems and policies

component of the environmental factors, the qualifiers denote the extent to which a certain factor is a facilitator or a barrier to the functioning of the person. Accordingly, the qualifier scale extends from +4 to –4.

According to the WHO, broad ranges of percentages are provided for those cases in which calibrated assessment instruments or other standards are available to quantify the impairment, activity limitation, participation restriction or environmental barrier/ facilitator. Table 2.4 shows the generic qualifier scale of the ICF. It is to be noted, that the generic qualifier scale is one option among others provided by the ICF, which also

Table 2.4   The generic International Classification of Functioning, Disability and Health (ICF) qualifier scale.

Qualifier	Description	
Functioning		Impairment, restriction, limitation, %
0	NO problem (none, absent, negligible...)	0–4
1	MILD problem (slight, low...)	5–24
2	MODERATE problem (medium, fair...)	25–49
3	SEVERE problem (high, extreme...)	50–95
4	COMPLETE problem (total...)	96–100
8	Not specified	
9	Not applicable	
Environmental factors		Barrier, facilitator
0	NO barrier or facilitator	0–4
1	MILD barrier	5–24
2	MODERATE barrier	25–49
3	SEVERE barrier	50–95
4	COMPLETE barrier	96–100
+1	MILD facilitator	5–24
+2	MODERATE facilitator	25–49
+3	SUBSTANTIAL facilitator	50–95
+4	COMPLETE facilitator	96–100
8	Barrier or facilitator: not specified	
9	Not applicable	

offers further options, especially for the coding of activities and participation, but also environmental factors. These further options are described in the ICF's Annex 2 and 3 (WHO, 2001).

2.3   The origins of the ICF

Models of disability help us in defining what disability is and how we can think and speak about it. The question 'what is disability?' is not new and the ICF was not the first approach to thinking about a model for disability. On the contrary, the ICF as a model can be viewed as the intermediate product of a 'quasi-evolutionary' development of disability models (Masala and Petretto, 2008; McDougall et al., 2010; Whiteneck, 2005). It integrates various lines of thought about disability into a 'meta-model'.

There are two principle strands of development that came together to form the ICF. The first has been called the 'medical model' derived from a concept of disability, which is that disability is the *consequence* of disease or injury in an individual. It should be noted that 'medical' in this sense does not necessarily refer to a single professional group, but to a way of thinking in which everything is explained by pathology (some kind of deviation from normal). The second strand is the 'social model', which considers that disability is primarily due to society's inability or difficulty in accommodating the particular needs and requirements of people with impairments.

The medical model strongly influenced the development of the WHO 1980 International Classification of Impairments, Disabilities and Handicaps (ICIDH) by Philip Wood, the precursor to the ICF (Kostanjsek et al., 2009). Possibly, the defining characteristic of the medical model is that disability is seen as a deficit of the individual, amenable to an 'expert' solution, leading to a restoration of optimal functioning to which all people aspire. For example, the definition of disability offered by Nagi (1964), which was highly congruent with the development of the ICIDH, was: 'Inability to engage in any substantial gainful activity by reason of a medically determinable impairment that is expected to be of long-continued and indefinite duration or to result in death' (Nagi, 1964).

It should be clearly noted that Nagi also recognized that 'inability' could be due to the environmental context alone, which presaged later developments of the ICF, but this original framework provided by Nagi distinguished the concepts of pathology, impairment, functional limitation and disability, which related to each other in a linear–causal way. This Functional Limitation Model became the most influential formulation of the biomedical understanding of disability over the following decades, and a number of subsequent models have built upon Nagi's framework, e.g. models by the Institutes of Medicine in the USA, the ICIDH-model of the WHO, the Disability Creation Process model of the Quebec Group in Canada (Fougeyrollas et al., 1998; Institute of Medicine et al., 1991, 1997; World Health Organization, 1980).

Viewed from this perspective, there is a linear, hierarchical progression of the consequences of pathology (Figure 2.2). The principal components of this model are conceived in negative terms; 'impairment' is a deficit of organ function, 'disability' is a deficit of functioning at the level of the whole person, 'handicap' is a deficit of functioning at the level of society.

Although this model represented a significant advance over a purely 'disease' based concept of health in which health equated with absence of disease, there are clearly many shortcomings. The nature of the language was seen as pejorative, the focus on a normative concept of disability conflicted significantly with a social model of disability and the idea that a linear, causal relationship exists between the components of the model was simplistic and inaccurate (Chatterji et al., 1999; Ustun et al., 1995). Nevertheless, the concept of separating out the manifestations of dysfunction by reference to the distinctions between organ (impairment), the whole organism (disability) and the organism's relation to other organisms (handicap) was fundamental and continues to inform current thinking about disability and health. This concept remains the crowning achievement of the ICIDH.

In contrast, the 'social model' of disability was generated outside of the health arena from the disability rights movement of the 1960s. The term itself appears to

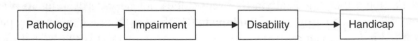

Figure 2.2   The International Classification of Impairments, Disabilities and Handicaps (ICIDH) model.

have first been used by Mike Oliver in 1983, to describe the view articulated by the UK Organisation Union of the Physically Impaired against Segregation (UPIAS), which was: 'In our view it is society which disables physically impaired people. Disability is something imposed on top of our impairments by the way we are unnecessarily isolated and excluded from full participation in society' (UPIAS, 1975).

From this perspective, disability is created by the failure of society to accommodate to the requirements of all its members (especially minority groups) rather than by failure of individuals to accommodate to the requirements of society. Whereas impairment might be related to health problems, disability only relates to society's response to those impairments. Hence, health (and the health professional) is largely irrelevant to the disabled person.

The biopsychosocial model brings these streams of thought together, although George Engel's original conception of the term in 1977 was influenced more by medicine's inappropriate reliance upon the biological sciences, especially molecular biology, than consideration of the phenomenon of disability (Engel, 1977). Yet the *systems theory approach* he proposed has been very influential upon the evolution of the ICIDH into the ICF, especially in moving away from a linear, cause and effect kind of thinking that solely focuses upon the body and disease: 'This approach, by treating sets of related events collectively as systems manifesting functions and properties on the specific level of the whole, has made possible recognition of isomorphies across different levels of organisation, as molecules, cells, organs, the organism, the person, the family, the society, or the biosphere' (Engel, 1977, p. 134).

The ICF does not go so far as to conceive of the biosphere, but the identification of the distinct elements of health conditions (pathology), body structures, body functions, activity limitations, participation restrictions, environmental factors and personal factors that may relate to each other in many different ways (these relationships are not assumed) is a systems approach to considering the concept of 'functioning'.

2.4 Using the ICF in practice – ICF core sets, rehabilitation cycle and ICF tools

Introduction

The ICF can be used in different settings and for various purposes, at individual and also at population levels, e.g. for research, health statistics, disability evaluation, education, and policy. In clinical rehabilitation, the ICF (WHO, 2001) can be applied together with the ICD to individuals with specific health conditions. The ICF is a highly comprehensive classification containing more than 1400 categories to describe people's functioning, disability and health. This comprehensiveness is a major advantage and strength of the ICF. But at the same time it is a major challenge to its practicability and feasibility.

For specific applications, especially in clinical practice, tailored tools need to be available, which simplify the use of the ICF and at the same time take advantage of its strengths. A number of such tools are currently available. First of all, the ICF core sets are named (these are discussed in detail in the following section), as they build the basis for further tools (Cieza et al., 2004a; Stucki et al., 2002, 2003). Further clinical ICF application tools are embedded in the model of the rehabilitation cycle: the ICF assessment sheet, the ICF categorical profile and evaluation display and the intervention table (Rauch et al., 2008, 2010a, 2010b; Steiner et al., 2002; Stucki et al., 2002; Swiss Paraplegic Research, 2007).

ICF core sets

The development of the ICF core sets is one approach to enhance the applicability of the ICF (Cieza et al., 2004a). This approach, in line with the underlying biopsycho-social model, explicitly connects functioning and disability categories, which are aetiologically neutral, to a defined health condition (or diagnosis) to facilitate data collection. The WHO has recognized that in everyday practice and in specific settings, only a fraction out of the total number of the ICF's categories is needed (Ustun et al., 2004). Thus, an ICF core set is a selection of categories out of the entire classification, which describe in a parsimonious way the functional impact of a certain specified health condition.

Scientifically based internationally agreed ICF core sets for a number of health conditions have been developed in WHO collaborative projects together with partner organizations worldwide. A selection of already available ICF core sets is listed in Table 2.5. For each of the health conditions two types of ICF core sets have been developed. Comprehensive ICF core sets include the prototypical spectrum of functioning problems in people with the given condition, to be used in multidisciplinary settings as a basis for comprehensive assessment and documentation. The brief ICF core sets serve in clinical encounters, but also in clinical and epidemiological studies or in health reporting, as minimum data-sets and represent a selection out of the corresponding comprehensive ICF core set. Using the universal terminology of the ICF, ICF core sets preserve all advantages and potentials of the classification as a common standard language, enhancing its feasibility at the same time by their manageable size.

The development of an ICF core set is an international process, conducted according to a standardized protocol in collaboration with WHO and partner organizations. The methodology integrates scientific evidence as well as consensus elements (Biering-Sorensen et al., 2006, ICF core set SCI). The development is basically a filtering process and consists overall of three phases: (1) preliminary studies, (2) consensus conference, and (3) validation and testing.

The preliminary studies use a triangulation approach and consider the consumer's perspective, the health professionals' and the clinical as well as the research perspective. The standard protocol includes qualitative focus group studies with service users, web-based expert surveys with health professionals from various disciplines, extensive empirical data collections using the ICF and systematic reviews of the literature. From these preliminary studies, a broad pool of ICF categories is pre-selected. The pre-selected categories are potential candidates to be included in the ICF core set.

Table 2.5 International Classification of Functioning, Disability and Health (ICF) core sets for specific health conditions.

ICF core sets	References
Ankylosing spondylitis (AS)	Boonen et al. (2010), ICF core set AS
Bipolar disorders	Vieta et al. (2007), ICF core set Bipolar
Breast cancer	Brach et al. (2004), ICF core set BC
Chronic ischemic heart disease (CIHD)	Cieza et al. (2004b), ICF core set CIHD
Chronic widespread pain (CWP)	Cieza et al. (2004c), ICF core set CWP; Hieblinger et al. (2009), ICF core set CWP
Depression	Cieza et al. (2004d), ICF core set Depression
Diabetes mellitus (DM)	Ruof et al. (2004), ICF core set DM; Kirchberger et al. (2009), ICF core set DM
Head and neck cancer (HNC)	Tschiesner et al. (2007), ICF core set HNC; Tschiesner et al. (2009), ICF core set HNC; Becker et al. (2010), ICF core set HNC; Tschiesner et al. (2010), ICF core set HNC
Low back pain (LBP)	Cieza et al. (2004e), ICF core set LBP; Roe et al. (2009), ICF core set LBP
Multiple sclerosis (MS)	Khan and Pallant (2007a, 2007b), ICF core set MS; Kesselring et al. (2008), ICF core set MS
Obesity	Stucki et al. (2004a), ICF core sets Obesity; Raggi et al. (2009), ICF core set Obesity
Obstructive pulmonary diseases (OPD)	Stucki et al. (2004b), ICF core set OPD; Rauch et al. (2009), ICF core set OPD
Osteoarthritis (OA)	Dreinhofer et al. (2004), ICF core set OA; Xie et al. (2007), ICF core set OA
Osteoporosis (OP)	Cieza et al. (2004f), ICF core set OP
Psoriasis	Taylor et al. (2010), ICF core set PsA
Psoriatic arthritis (PsA)	Taylor et al. (2010), ICF core set PsA
Rheumatoid arthritis (RA)	Stucki et al. (2004c), ICF core set RA; Coenen et al. (2006), ICF core set RA; Kirchberger et al. (2007), ICF core set RA; Uhlig et al. (2007), ICF core set RA; Uhlig et al. (2009), ICF core set RA
Sleep disorders	Gradinger et al. (2009), ICF core set Sleep
Spinal cord injury (SCI)	Biering-Sorensen et al. (2006), ICF core set SCI; Cieza et al. (2010), ICF core set SCI; Kirchberger et al. (2010), ICF core set SCI
Stroke	Geyh et al. (2004), ICF core set Stroke; Starrost et al. (2008), ICF core set Stroke; Alguren et al. (2010), ICF core set Stroke; Lemberg et al. (2010), ICF core set Stroke
Systemic lupus erythematosis & systemic sclerosis	Aringer et al. (2006), ICF core set Lupus
Traumatic brain injury (TBI)	Aiachini et al. (2010), ICF core set TBI

The ICF categories, which resulted from the phase 1 preliminary studies, enter the consensus process. In phase 2, for each health condition, an international consensus conference takes place with representatively selected experts from different world regions and different professional backgrounds. The consensus conference follows a

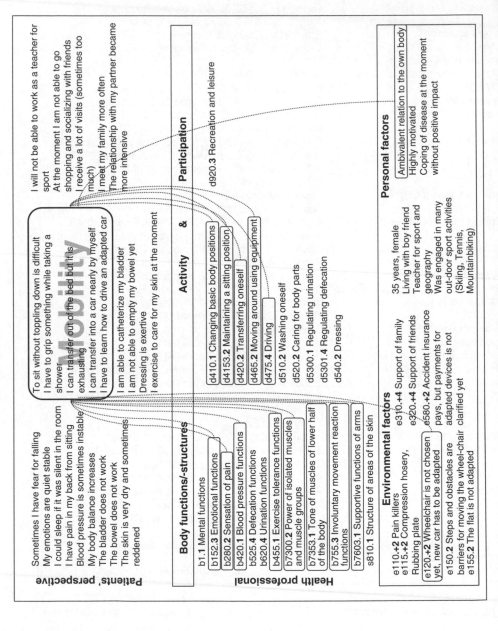

Figure 2.3 International Classification of Functioning, Disability and Health (ICF) assessment sheet. The ICF codes in the health professional's section are composed of the ICF category and the ICF qualifier (marked here in bold). (Designed by and reproduced with permission from William Levack.)

structured nominal group process with discussion and voting rounds according to predefined procedures and decision criteria. The comprehensive and the brief ICF core sets are the final output of phase 2. These short lists of ICF categories to be used in a certain health condition are validated and tested in phase 3, in national as well as international efforts from different perspectives. Phase 3 is an open-ended process that continuously provides information to the users about the ICF core sets in various settings.

The rehabilitation cycle and ICF tools

Although Chapter 4 discusses the rehabilitation cycle in more detail, we will consider specifically how the ICF fits into each stage of the cycle. The ICF tools to be used in clinical rehabilitation management utilize the ICF core sets. The ICF tools serve to enhance assessment and documentation, implementation, management as well as evaluation of rehabilitation services. For the rehabilitation team, the ICF tools serve to enhance their everyday tasks, which include information exchange and multidisciplinary communication, intervention coordination, documentation and reporting (Rauch et al., 2008, 2010a, 2010b; Swiss Paraplegic Research, 2007). The ICF tools are embedded in the rehabilitation-cycle model (Steiner et al., 2002; Stucki et al., 2002). The rehabilitation cycle is a cybernetic model and views rehabilitation as a clearly structured and iterative problem-solving process. The process includes four steps: (1) assessment (2) goal setting, (3) intervention and (4) evaluation (see Chapter 4, Figure 4.1).

The ICF assessment sheet

The ICF assessment sheet is a one-page overview of an individual's functioning and disability status, based on the ICF's biopsychosocial model. It is typically completed at the interdisciplinary team conference after the first assessment of the person by all involved professionals has been concluded.

The ICF assessment sheet summarizes the service-user perspective as well as the health professional team's perspective on the body level of functioning problems, activity limitations and participation restrictions. In addition, the environmental and personal factors are relevant.

The service-user's perspective is displayed on the upper section of the sheet by using the person's own words to describe their individual experience. The health professionals' perspective is reflected on the lower part of the sheet. All results from the clinical assessments relevant to the description of the actual functioning status are summarized using the standardized and common language of the ICF categories. As an alternative, it is also possible to use the original technical terminology of the health professionals along with the ICF terminology. Figure 2.3 shows an example of an ICF assessment sheet for a person with spinal cord injury.

The ICF categorical profile

The ICF categorical profile (Figure 2.4) is an illustration of the functioning status of a person with a health condition at the time of assessment. The profile is created using

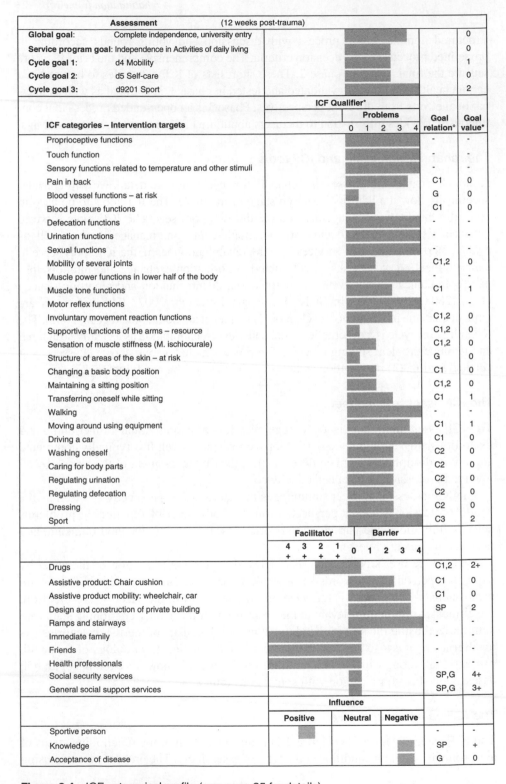

Figure 2.4 ICF categorical profile (see page 25 for details)

the categories of the according comprehensive ICF core set. For each of the ICF categories relevant in the given case, the qualifier values are rated based on information gathered by the rehabilitation professionals and is depicted in the form of a horizontal histogram. Thus, a profile of the severity of the person's functioning difficulties is produced. The profile provides information to identify targets for interventions, to set and monitor intervention goals.

The ICF intervention table

The ICF intervention table (Figure 2.5) contains those ICF categories that have been identified as targets for rehabilitation intervention, structured according to the model components: body functions and structures, activity and participation, environmental and personal factors. The table includes the intervention that is to be conducted and the health professional disciplines involved. At the same time, the initial qualifier for the severity of the functioning problems, the goal value in this domain, as well as the achieved value, is also documented in the intervention table. Thus, the changes during the course of interventions can be monitored. Information from the ICF categorical profile and/or the ICF assessment sheet helps to create the ICF intervention table.

The ICF evaluation display

The ICF evaluation display (Figure 2.6) is a pre–post intervention depiction of the ICF categorical profile. It lists the rehabilitation goals and intervention targets in terms of ICF categories and displays the profile of functioning status at initial assessment. Along with this, it also shows the outcomes of the interventions by the end of the rehabilitation cycle, again in the form of a profile. The display pictures clearly the changes in the functioning status after treatment. Goal achievement for each of the ICF categories is also documented in a simple yes/no or plus/minus format. Based on the ICF evaluation display the rehabilitation team discusses and decides together with the service user if the initiation of a further rehabilitation cycle with new or modified goals is necessary and promising, or if the person should be referred to a successive service programme, or if the rehabilitation intervention should be ended.

Figure 2.4   International Classification of Functioning, Disability and Health (ICF) categorical profile: extraction. Illustrates the aspects of the functioning status that are relevant for this patient (Spinal cord injury, ASIA A Th 3).

*ICF qualifier range from 0 = no problem to 4 = complete problem In the components of body functions (b), body structures (s), activity and participation (d) and from −4 = complete barrier to +4 = complete facilitator in the environmental factors. In personal factors, the sign + and − indicates to what extent a determined personal factor has a positive or negative influence on the individual's functioning.

°C1,2,3 mark the relation to cycle goals 1, 2, 3; SG is related to service programme goal, G is related to the global goal.

Intervention target		Intervention	Doctor	Nurse	PT / Spo	OT	Psychology	Social worker	Arch	First value	Goal value	End value
Body functions/structures	b28013 Pain in the back	Body posture training	☐	☐	⊠	☐	☐	☐	☐			
		Adaptation of wheelchair	☐	☐	☐	⊠	☐	☐	☐	3	0	1
		Control of sitting position	☐	⊠	⊠	⊠	☐	☐	☐			
		Medication	⊠	⊠	☐	☐	☐	☐	☐			
	b415 Blood vessel functions – at risk	Compression hosery, drugs	⊠	⊠	☐	☐	☐	☐	☐	0	0	0
	b420 Blood pressure function	Compression hosery	⊠	⊠	☐	☐	☐	☐	☐	1	0	0
	b7101 Mobility of several joints	Passive movement	☐	☐	⊠	☐	☐	☐	⊠	1	0	1
	b755 Involuntary movement functions	Body balance–training	☐	☐	⊠	☐	☐	☐	☐	2	0	0
	b7800 Sensation of muscle stiffness	Detonisation, Stretching	☐	⊠	☐	☐	☐	☐	☐	1	0	0
	s810 Structure of the skin – at risk	Daily inspection	☐	⊠	☐	☐	☐	☐	☐	0	0	0
Activities and Participation	d410 Changing basic body positions	Sit-up-training	☐	☐	⊠	☐	☐	☐	☐	1	0	0
	d4153 Maintaining in a sitting position	Body balance training	☐	☐	⊠	☐	☐	☐	☐	1	0	0
	d4200 Transferring oneself while sitting	Transfer-training	☐	☐	⊠	⊠	☐	☐	☐	2	1	1
	d465 Moving around with wheelchair	Wheelchair-training outdoor	☐	☐	⊠	☐	☐	☐	☐	3	1	2
	d510 Washing oneself	Assistance/Instruction	☐	⊠	☐	☐	☐	☐	☐	2	0	0
	d520 Caring for body parts	Assistance/Instruction	☐	⊠	☐	☐	☐	☐	☐	2	0	1
	d5300 Regulating urination	Assistance/Instruction	☐	⊠	☐	☐	☐	☐	☐	2	0	0
	d5301 Regulating defecation	Assistance/Instruction	☐	⊠	☐	⊠	☐	☐	☐	2	0	0
	d540 Dressing	Assistance/Instruction	☐	⊠	☐	☐	☐	☐	☐	2	0	0
	d9201 Sport	Exercising different sports	☐	☐	⊠	☐	☐	☐	☐	4	2	2

EF	e1151 Assistive products: Chair cushion	Control of chair cushion	□	□	□	☒	□	□	□	−2	0	0
	e1201 Assistive products for personal mobility: Wheelchair and adapted car	Testing of different wheelchairs, Reconstruction of car	□	□	□	☒	□	□	□	−3	−2	−2
	e155 Design, construction and building products and technology of buildings for private use: farmer house	Planning and reconstruction of private building	□	□	□	☒	□	□	☒	−3	−2	−2
	e5700 Social security services	Clarification, Organisation of payments	□	□	□	□	□	☒	□	0	4+	2+
PF	Knowledge	Teaching, consulting and lectures	☒	☒	☒	☒	□	□	□	2	2+	2+
	Acceptance/Coping of disease	Behavioral training approaches	□	☒	☒	☒	□	□	□	1	0	1+

Figure 2.5 International Classification of Functioning, Disability and Health (ICF) intervention table: spinal cord injury.

Arch, Architect (spinal cord injury, ASIA A Th 3, 12 weeks after trauma).

EF, environmental factors; OT, occupational therapy; PF, personal factors; PT, physiotherapy; Spo, sports physiotherapy.

Assessment	(12 weeks post-trauma)
Global goal:	Complete independence, university entry
Service program goal:	Independence in Activities of daily living
Cycle goal 1:	d4 Mobility
Cycle goal 2:	d5 Self-care
Cycle goal 3:	d9201 Sport

Evaluation	(16 weeks post-trauma)
Cycle goal 1:	not evaluated yet
Cycle goal 2:	not evaluated yet

Code	ICF categories – Intervention targets	ICF qualifier* Problems (0–4)	Goal relation°	Goal value*	ICF qualifier* Problems (0–4)	Goal achievement
b28013	Pain in back		1	0		-
b415	Blood vessel functions – at risk		G	0		✓
b420	Blood pressure functions		1	0		✓
b7101	Mobility of several joints		1,2	0		-
b735	Muscle tone functions		1	1		✓
b755	Involuntary movement reaction functions		1,2	0		✓
b7603	Supportive functions of the arms – resource		1,2	0		✓
b7800	Sensation of muscle stiffness (M. ischiocurale)		1,2	0		✓
s810	Structure of areas of the skin – at risk		G	0		✓
d410	Changing a basic body position		1	0		✓
d4153	Maintaining a sitting position		1,2	0		✓
d4200	Transferring oneself while sitting		1	1		✓
d465	Moving around using equipment		1	1		-
d4751	Driving a car		1	0		✓
d510	Washing oneself		2	0		✓
d520	Caring for body parts		2	0		-
d5300	Regulating urination		2	0		✓
d5301	Regulating defecation		2	0		✓
d540	Dressing		2	0		✓
d9201	Sport		3	2		✓

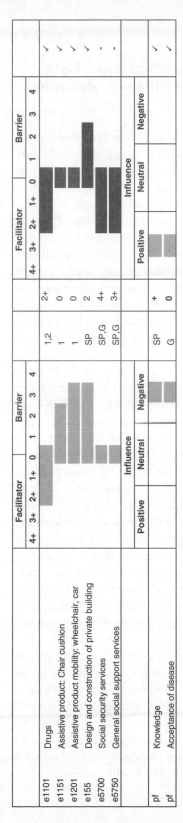

Figure 2.6 International Classification of Functioning, Disability and Health (ICF) evaluation display: illustrates the change of the functioning status over the course of one cycle (Spinal Cord Injury, ASIA A Th 3, 12 and 16 weeks after trauma).

* ICF qualifier range from 0 = no problem to 4 = complete problem in the components of body functions (b), body structures (s), activity and participation (d) and from –4 = complete barrier to +4 = complete facilitator in the environmental factors. In personal factors, the sign + and – indicates to what extent a determined personal factor has a positive or negative influence on the individual's functioning.

° 1,2,3 mark the relation to cycle goals 1, 2, 3; SG is related to service programme goal, G is related to the global goal.

2.5 Can the ICF be used to measure functioning – both the 'what' and the 'how'? Controversies – to measure or to classify that is the question

Although the ICF is a widely accepted model and a sound basis for rehabilitation management (Gutenbrunner et al., 2007), certain aspects about the model, the classification and its implementation are matters of dispute. One of the issues, which arise in relation to the practical application of the ICF is the issue of operationalization and measurement. The ICF is a classification, but is used with the qualifier scales to describe the severity of problems in the different areas of functioning. Thus, the ICF is sometimes confused with a questionnaire or rating scale. Nevertheless, the ICF is still not a measurement instrument but a classification. Measurement and classification are two different approaches towards the description of individual's burden, functioning and health. The two approaches can be regarded as complementary but distinct. Although from the classification perspective the ICF and the ICF core sets serve as standards to define *what* to measure, from the perspective of health status measurement the question *how* to measure is not addressed. The 'how to measure' question is more fully addressed in Chapter 5.

The ICF provides a guide for measurement, a means to systematically organize results of assessments, a means to systematically organize clinical judgement and to create a compatible informational base for different purposes. The key difference between a measure and a classification tool is that a classification serves as the reference among different measurement instruments at different facilities, and even in different countries, thus being the framework and organizing principle where all information can flow together into the same common system. This means that a classification-based tool can be used to organize qualitative information (e.g. 'How are you doing today, Mrs Jones?') as well as quantitative information (e.g. Life Satisfaction Scale scores (LISAT), Fugl-Meyer et al., 1991), results of observer-rated (e.g. Functional Independence Measure, Granger et al., 1993) and self-reported (e.g. Visual Analogue Scale for pain) scales, physical measures (e.g. grip strength dynamometer) and questionnaire scores (e.g. Hand Function domain of the Stroke Impact Scale, Duncan et al., 1999), and so on. The current use of the ICF, the ICF core sets and the ICF tools relies on clinical judgements combining different kinds of available information (observation, interviews, measurements and records), summarizing them into one qualifier per ICF category.

In the literature, measurement is sometimes seen as a contrast or alternative to classification. However, it is important to note: to measure or to classify, that is not the question. Just as in medical diagnostics, where anamnestic information, physical examination, results of laboratory tests, imaging techniques, etc. are combined into a diagnosis and expressed in terms of the ICD code, the quantitative results of rehabilitation assessments are the objects that enter the ICF classification. The classification represents the ordering principle and the structure to summarize, store, retrieve, and convey different kinds of information about people's functioning, disability and health.

The question that arises is how the measurement and the classification approach can be connected with each other. For the connection of the measurement and the classification approach, basically two strategies can be followed. Existing measures can be linked with the ICF, or, operationalizations and measures based on the ICF can be developed.

The ICF has been used recently in systematic literature reviews of measurement instruments applying the ICF model (e.g. Salter et al., 2005a, 2005b, 2005c) or the ICF classification (using 'linking rules', Cieza and Stucki, 2005; Cieza et al., 2002, 2005; Geyh et al., 2007; Post et al., 2010). The results of these kinds of analyses of measures in the light of the classification, are helpful to connect the ICF with the instruments that are widely used in clinical and research practice. One step further along this road are some first attempts that have already been undertaken to connect the scores that result from questionnaire types of assessments with the ICF qualifier scale using Rasch analyses techniques (Cieza et al., 2009).

Also from the very beginnings of the ICIDH and the ICF, some instrument developers have used the model and the classification as a framework for health-status instruments. Numerous instruments have been created based on the ICF and the ICIDH, such as the WHODAS (WHO, 2000), IMPACT (Post et al., 2008), the Burden of Stroke Scale (Doyle et al., 2004) or the Stroke Impact Scale (Duncan et al., 1999). However, there is an unmet need for measures that are consistent with the ICF as a model and as a classification, as well as for developing algorithms that make the relationship between different measures and the classification explicit to enhance the objectivity of the qualifier scaling and to facilitate the implementation of the ICF in everyday clinical practice.

2.6 Controversies – classification of 'participation restrictions' versus 'activity limitations'

Case studies

Ralph is a 77-year-old man with many health problems including congestive heart failure from ischaemic heart disease, osteoarthritis and diabetes. He lives with his wife who also has health problems but is generally the healthier of the two. In all their married life, Ralph has been responsible for cooking the Sunday dinner – a large affair that members of their family generally attend. In recent months, he has found it more difficult to produce the Sunday dinner and he has needed to accept help from his wife, which he feels unhappy about.

Jessica is a 32-year-old woman who used to work as an insurance broker. She suffered a traumatic brain injury after falling from her bicycle while not wearing a helmet. She has not been able to return to work and although is living alone, requires assistance from social services to prepare most evening meals and to assist with other household activities.

According to the ICF classification system, difficulties with preparing a major meal would be coded as *d6301 Preparing complex meals*. This code does not tell us whether the problem is an activity limitation or a participation restriction. In fact, the ICF classification does not differentiate between activities and participation at all but lists all such domains within a single component distributed across nine chapters. For Ralph, where preparing a meal is somewhat of a life role, it is fair to judge that his difficulty is a participation restriction. For Jessica, where the salience and social context of preparing meals is quite different, it is plausible to consider her difficulty as an activity limitation.

The rationale for amalgamating activities and participation into a single list and not distinguishing between them is obscure and is somewhat incongruous with the ICF model. Annex 3 of the ICF classification manual (WHO, 2001) does suggest four possible approaches to indicate the specificity of categories under the activities and participation component, but there is little guidance as to the most appropriate. The suggested approaches are as follows.

1 Consider the first four chapters as activities (learning and applying knowledge, general tasks and demands, communication, mobility) and the second four chapters as participation (self-care, domestic life, interpersonal interactions, major life areas, community and civic life).
2 Consider a partial overlap whereby categories with the chapters communication, mobility, self-care and domestic life could be considered either activity or participation depending on context.
3 Consider first- and second-level categories as participation and deeper level categories as activities.
4 All categories could be considered activity and participation and could be coded twice as to each perspective.

The last suggestion was the approach taken by Eide and colleagues (2008), which was to consider an activity limitation to be a question of *capacity*, that is, the extent to which a person had difficulty with a task given an ideal and perfectly accommodating environment, whereas participation restriction is a question of *performance*, that is, the extent to which a person had difficulty with the same task in his/her ordinary living environment. In quantifying the extent of activity limitations and participation restrictions in this way, factor analysis was shown to lead to largely the same ICF categories loading on dimensions of participation, as loading on dimensions of activities, suggesting that the capacity–performance paradigm alone does little to distinguish between the concepts of activity and participation.

None of these approaches have been universally endorsed and calls for resolution of the operational differentiation between the two concepts of activities and participation have been made by bodies as important as the US Institute of Medicine. There have been several suggestions about how to resolve the problem but mostly the proposals are not fully successful and tend to conflict with each other. Whiteneck and Dijkers (2009) propose a return to some of the concepts of the ICIDH by considering that the defining characteristics of participation are that (1) it represents the societal perspective; (2) it encompasses the notion of social role performance; (3) it may involve 'building blocks' of activities but that the composition of these blocks may be quite different to build the same role; (4) it is a relational concept that makes sense only in a particular context, whereas activities are characteristics of individual people.

Using these characteristics and taking the example of Ralph and Jessica, it is thus clear that being responsible for the family Sunday meal represents participation whereas merely preparing a meal is an activity. It is possible for Ralph to be responsible for the Sunday dinner without actually doing the cooking – the role could plausibly continue but put together with a different series of activities, for instance he could direct proceedings, teach a grandchild his particular methods, prepare the menu, order the food online or by telephone and preside at the table. Preparing a meal then, is seen as an activity that may (but not necessarily) be part of a social role. For Jessica, living alone, there is no relational aspect to preparing meals. The activity has little or no social salience and her difficulty is an individual characteristic. Making the distinction is often clinically important. Training to assist Jessica to prepare meals is a sensible and direct route to improving her ability and independence but this may or may not be a useful intervention for Ralph, once the full context of the situation is understood.

Measurement of the two concepts also requires that the distinctions are properly appreciated and the concepts are precisely conceived. Measurement of activity limitations is reasonably straightforward and there are many questionnaires and scales to help quantify this concept. However, measurement of participation restrictions, even when precisely understood is very problematic and may not be possible in terms similar to the quantification of activity limitations.

A critical issue as to whether participation can be quantified is that the concept is probably non-hierarchical. This poses difficulties in producing a number (quantity) that properly represents the concept on a meaningful scale. For example, a participation measure might include items related to employment, going to the movies, voting in elections, attending church or being a student. It is quite uncertain whether difficulties with these items can be sensibly ranked in order of least to most participation. Without an ordinal nature to the items on a scale, summation of item scores is nonsensical. This is a different situation to activity limitations, where task difficulty across different tasks can usually be ordered sensibly from least to most difficult.

Furthermore, the complexity of participation domains suggests the strong possibility of multiple dimensions. It may be more logical to develop subscales for different aspects of participation represented by the different level 1 categories (chapter headings) of the ICF. Whiteneck (2010) provides a detailed review of the difficulties of participation measurement and makes some suggestions for a way forward (this article is strongly recommended for readers who wish to pursue participation measurement in research settings).

For clinicians (and others), who wish to determine outcomes expressed in participation terms, traditional indicators such as percentage of people returning to work or to live in non-institutional care, or who are economically self-sufficient remain reasonable (albeit blunt) markers.

2.7 Controversies – is the ICF a framework for understanding 'QoL'?

> **Case study**
>
> Jack is a 27-year-old man with schizophrenia. He was recently discharged from hospital after an exacerbation of psychosis, back to live with his parents, whom he distrusts and dislikes. When living in the environment of a flat, he eats erratically, has poor personal hygiene and sometimes forgets to pay bills. His parents maintain that that the QoL for Jack is much better when living with them since he is well cared for and he leads a more regulated lifestyle. However, Jack is much more interested in living in a flat and quickly leaves home after only 2 days. He says that his QoL is better when he is on his own.

The meaning of the term 'quality of life' is difficult to pin down precisely, yet it is popular as an end-point of clinical trials and to inform public policy. Part of the attraction of the concept may be its universality, in that enhancements to QoL can only ever be positive, and that QoL measurement might appear to provide a common metric (single index) with which to evaluate diverse health or social projects. Many of the components of the ICF, particularly the notion of participation, and categories within the activities and participation chapters, are also present in many questionnaires that purport to measure health-related QoL. However, as it is currently construed, the ICF is designed to determine the level of functioning (across various components) and is explicitly not concerned with how people *feel* about that level of functioning.

In the case study, Jack does not function very well when he is on his own, particularly from the point of view of his parents. When assessed by the ICF, he would also be rated as having difficulties with self-care activities that would not be so apparent when living in a more supervised environment. However, he has a different opinion about what matters. His QoL is not adequately represented by the ICF because the ICF only takes into account the degree to which certain functions are problematic, but not whether these problems actually matter to the person concerned. That the current format of the ICF is not explicitly related to QoL is a criticism that can also be levelled at many other self-report questionnaires that purport to measure health-related QoL (HRQoL). In its favour, the ICF has never claimed this property whereas some other questionnaires are commonly reported as measuring HRQoL. Foremost among these is the Short Form-36 (SF-36). Although this is referred to as a health survey by its developers rather than as a measure of HRQoL, it is very commonly reported as such. Similarly to the ICF, the SF-36 contains no items that ask respondents how they feel about any negatively scored item. Personal perception of one's life circumstances is a critically important component of QoL; without this component, only health status is being assessed.

Having said that perception of one's life circumstances is a critical component of HRQoL, it is important to note that there is no broadly accepted theoretical model for

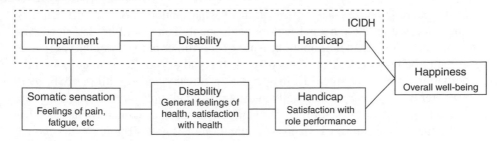

Figure 2.7 Integration of the International Classification of Impairments, Disabilities and Handicaps (ICIDH) with a concept of health-related quality of life. (Post et al., 1999, reproduced with permission from Sage Publications)

HRQoL. A large number of concepts have been used to measure QoL including objective indicators, subjective indicators, satisfaction of human needs, psychological models, health and functioning models, social health models, social cohesion and social capital, environmental models and ideographic models. These are reviewed in some detail by Brown and colleagues (2004).

There have been two interesting proposals that integrate the ICF with notions of QoL. Pre-dating the ICF, was a model proposed by Post and colleagues in 1999 that considered the ICIDH rather than the ICF (Figure 2.7). However, the approach is equally applicable to the ICF in that it considers the person's perceptions of each major component of functioning, which could be integrated into an overall sense of well-being (happiness).

An operationalization of this approach is described by the authors of the Utrecht Scale for Evaluation of Rehabilitation – Participation (USER-P). In this self-report measure, the 31 items (covering eight of the nine ICF activities and participation chapters) are divided into three groups: (1) frequency of participation, (2) restrictions with participation and (3) satisfaction with participation (van der Zee et al., 2010). Each group is scored separately, thus allowing identification of level of functioning but also level of satisfaction with that level of functioning. However, the final step in the model of Figure 2.7 is not taken – each of the three scores of USER-P is presented separately and not integrated.

A more recent and ingenious second proposal uses the new component of *personal factors* of the ICF to incorporate the concepts of personal perceptions, meaningfulness, aspiration and intention. In this way, personal perception of one's health condition could be included within the ICF framework (Huber et al., 2010). The component of personal factors represents a major and radical evolution from the ICIDH to the ICF. This is reflected somewhat by the fact that personal factors have not yet been classified and that the precise boundaries of this component are still being discovered. It is unclear whether the ICF should include subjective judgements, or only levels of functioning (Ueda and Okawa, 2003). Huber et al. (2010) argue that personal factors could potentially include personal perceptions and not just 'objectively assessed' personal factors that are not classified elsewhere. This proposal is rather interesting from a conceptual and also practical perspective.

In the example above, Jack's perception of what matters most to him could be encapsulated within the personal factors component. This could be described as a sense of autonomy, self-determination, sense of control, or probably in his case, more specifically being independent of his parents. It could also be considered within the participation component since 'Human rights' is already coded with the ICF: *d940 Human rights* 'Enjoying all nationally and internationally recognized rights that are accorded to people by virtue of their humanity alone, such as human rights as recognized by the United Nations Universal Declaration of Human Rights (1948) and the United Nations Standard Rules for the Equalization of Opportunities for Persons with Disabilities (1993); the right to self-determination or autonomy; and the right to control over one's destiny'(WHO, 2001).

However, when considering the situation from a QoL perspective, it is not the level of d940 that is important but the satisfaction to which the individual accords that level. If Jack was not really bothered by being under the direct supervision of his parents but living in chaos was troubling, then he would have the same level of d940 by living in a flat alone, but less QoL. The key difference is how he feels about things. How would that be represented within the personal factors component? The approach of Huber and colleagues' would be to consider the concepts of meaningfulness, aspiration and intention with regards to the levels of functioning contained within the other ICF components. Thus, Jack imbues self-determination with especially high meaningfulness (perhaps to the exclusion of other healthy behaviours), aspires to achieve self-determination and takes action to achieve this aspiration.

2.8 Future developments of the ICF

In comparison with other members of the WHO Family of International Classifications (FIC), especially its older sibling the ICD, the ICF is in its infancy, having been first released in 2001, its history starting with the ICIDH published in 1980. The ICD has a history of more than 100 years and is currently undergoing its 11th revision. Similarly, it can be expected that the ICF will further develop, and undergo update and revision.

The ICF mentions several steps to further enhance the ICF emphasizing thereby the application perspective and the adaptation to the needs of different users. These steps include especially the use of the ICF in clinical and research settings, in health statistics, the development of eligibility algorithms for social benefits and pension, computerized applications, and assessment instruments (WHO, 2001, p. 250). Also the Institute of Medicine has stated a number of issues for the further development of the ICF, mainly from a conceptual point of view (Institute of Medicine et al., 1997, 2007).

The controversies addressed earlier in this chapter, including operationalization and measurement, harmonizing activities and participation as well as the relation of the ICF conceptualization to the important constructs of QoL and HRQoL, are certainly major issues for further discussion and for inclusion in the upcoming update process from the conceptual point of view. In addition, the issue of specifying the classification of environmental factors in more detail is a frequent call. The newly developed ICF-CY (Children and Youth), which specifically amends the ICF categories and definitions by aspects important for applicability across all age groups, is going to be considered as well (WHO, 2007).

However, one of the main challenges in the further development of the ICF is the amendment of the yet missing component of personal factors. The ICF states that these have not been developed for reasons of cultural diversity associated with them. But more pragmatic reasons might have also played a role in the decision to publish the ICF without the development of this component. The ICF characterizes personal factors as follows:

> Personal Factors are the particular background of an individual's life and living, and comprise features of the individual that are not part of a health condition or health states. These factors may include gender, race, age, other health conditions, fitness, lifestyle, habits, upbringing, coping styles, social background, education, profession, past and current experience (past life events and concurrent events), overall behaviour pattern and character style, individual psychological assets and other characteristics, all or any of which may play a role in disability at any level' (WHO, 2001).

The personal factors component of the ICF responds to the obvious and fundamental fact that people are different as individuals. These differences need to be taken into account in considering functioning, disability and health. The provision of best care, respecting individuality, autonomy and dignity of the person, understanding and explaining the current health state of the person, all require knowledge about the individual. A personal factors component responds to the question as to who the affected individuals are, where they stand in their lives, how they think and feel, what they want and how they usually manage themselves. Person-centred service delivery at stages of the rehabilitation process (Gutenbrunner et al., 2007; Steiner et al., 2002), especially individualized tailored interventions and shared decision making, but also epidemiological research, health reporting, and administration, rely on information about personal factors.

The development of the personal factors classification is currently under consideration by the WHO. Indeed, a number of challenges are associated with the development of this specific component. The first issue is the conceptualization of personal factors, which has to be in line with the ICF and non-overlapping with body functions and structures (especially mental functions), activities and participation, or the environmental factors. On the side of formal and methodological issues, the classification structure itself needs to be developed to contain mutually exclusive and jointly exhaustive categories. It needs to be backed up by a rigorous scientific development process, cross-cultural applicability testing as well as international agreement involving people with disabilities. Furthermore, the development process needs to adhere to WHO FIC standards to be endorsed by the WHO (Jacob et al., 2007; Madden et al., 2007).

Considering the conceptualization of personal factors, ICF experts from all over the world have thought about the personal factors component and some have already made first attempts and suggestions as how to structure the classification (Badley, 2006; Heerkens et al., 2004; Stephens and Kerr, 2000; Ueda and Okawa, 2003; Viol et al., 2006). In comparing these suggestions, certain common elements can be identified and can be taken as a rough preview on how a future classification might be structured. Three different parts emerge: one part on sociodemographic factors (e.g. age, gender, nationality, etc), a second part on elements of subjective experience (e.g. feelings, thoughts and motives) and a third part addressing objective descriptors of a person's behavioural patterns and styles (e.g. styles of self-management, coping strategies, personality traits).

Harmonizing, elaborating, and testing the classification of personal factors is going to be an exciting major step adding to the usefulness of the ICF and broadening its potential for multidisciplinary and consumer-centred practical applications, improving interventions and services for people with disabilities, and strengthening the individual's perspective in the ICF.

Additional resources

The ICF by web-browser can be accessed at:
http://apps.who.int/classifications/icfbrowser/ (accessed 5 March 2012).

The ICF Research Branch has a wealth of information about the ICF available online. For example, there is an eLearning-Module to learn more about the ICF:
http://www.icf-research-branch.org/ (accessed 5 March 2012).

To learn about the ICF and the clinical implementation of the ICF tools, visit:
http://www.icf-casestudies.org/ (accessed 5 March 2012).

References

Aiachini, B., Pisoni, C., Cieza, A., Cazzulani, B., Giustini, A. and Pistarini, C. (2010). Developing ICF core set for subjects with traumatic brain injury: an Italian clinical perspective. *European Journal of Physical and Rehabilitation Medicine*, *46*(1), 27–36.

Alguren, B., Lundgren-Nilsson, A. and Sunnerhagen, K. S. (2010). Functioning of stroke survivors–A validation of the ICF core set for stroke in Sweden. *Disability and Rehabilitation*, *32*(7), 551–559.

Aringer, M., Stamm, T. A., Pisetsky, D. S., Yarboro, C. H., Cieza, A., Smolen, J. S. and Stucki, G. (2006). ICF core sets: how to specify impairment and function in systemic lupus erythematosus. *Lupus*, *15*(4), 248–253.

Badley, E. M. (2006). More than facilitators and barriers: fitting the full range of environmental and personal contextual factors into the ICF model. *Proceedings of the Twelfth Annual North American Collaborating Centre Conference on ICF*. Vancouver, June 5–7. http://secure.cihi.ca/cihiweb/en/downloads/Elizabeth%20Badley%20-%20Looking%20Ahead.pdf (accessed 5 March 2012).

Becker, S., Kirchberger, I., Cieza, A., Berghaus, A., Harreus, U., Reichel, O. and Tschiesner, U. (2010). Content validation of the Comprehensive ICF core set for head and neck cancer (HNC): the perspective of psychologists. *Psychooncology*, *19*(6), 594–605.

Biering-Sorensen, F., Scheuringer, M., Baumberger, M., Charlifue, S. W., Post, M. W., Montero, F. and Stucki, G. (2006). Developing core sets for persons with spinal cord injuries based on the International Classification of Functioning, Disability and Health as a way to specify functioning. *Spinal Cord*, *44*(9), 541–546.

Boonen, A., Braun, J., van der Horst Bruinsma, I. E., Huang, F., Maksymowych, W., Kostanjsek, N. and van der Heijde, D. (2010). ASAS/WHO ICF core sets for ankylosing spondylitis (AS): how to classify the impact of AS on functioning and health. *Annals of the Rheumatic Diseases*, *69*(1), 102–107.

Boorse, C. (1975). On the distinction between disease and illness. *Philosophy and Public Affairs*, *5*(1), 49–68.

Boorse, C. (1977). Health as a theoretical concept. *Philosophy of Science*, *44*(4), 542–573.

Brach, M., Cieza, A., Stucki, G., Fussl, M., Cole, A., Ellerin, B. and Melvin, J. (2004). ICF core sets for breast cancer. *Journal of Rehabilitation Medicine*, *44*(Supplement), 121–127.

Brown, J., Bowling, A. and Flynn, T. (2004). *Models of Quality of Life: A Taxonomy, Overview and Systematic Review of the Literature*. Sheffield: European Forum and Population Aging Research. http://www.ageingresearch.group.shef.ac.uk/pdf/qol_review_complete.pdf (accessed 5 October 2011).

Chatterji, S., Ustun, B. and Bickenbach, J. E. (1999). What is disability after all? *Disability and Rehabilitation*, *21*(8), 396–398.

Cieza, A. and Stucki, G. (2005). Content comparison of health-related quality of life (HRQOL) instruments based on the international classification of functioning, disability and health (ICF). *Quality of Life Research*, *14*(5), 1225–1237.

Cieza, A., Brockow, T., Ewert, T., Amman, E., Kollerits, B., Chatterji, S. and Stucki, G. (2002). Linking health-status measurements to the international classification of functioning, disability and health. *Journal of Rehabilitation Medicine*, *34*(5), 205–210.

Cieza, A., Ewert, T., Ustun, T. B., Chatterji, S., Kostanjsek, N. and Stucki, G. (2004a). Development of ICF core sets for patients with chronic conditions. *Journal of Rehabilitation Medicine*, *44*(Supplement), 9–11.

Cieza, A., Stucki, A., Geyh, S., Berteanu, M., Quittan, M., Simon, A. and Walsh, N. (2004b). ICF core sets for chronic ischaemic heart disease. *Journal of Rehabilitation Medicine*, *44*(Supplement), 94–99.

Cieza, A., Stucki, G., Weigl, M., Kullmann, L., Stoll, T., Kamen, L. and Walsh, N. (2004c). ICF core sets for chronic widespread pain. *Journal of Rehabilitation Medicine*, *44*(Supplement), 63–68.

Cieza, A., Chatterji, S., Andersen, C., Cantista, P., Herceg, M., Melvin, J. and de Bie, R. (2004d). ICF core sets for depression. *Journal of Rehabilitation Medicine*, *44*(Supplement), 128–134.

Cieza, A., Stucki, G., Weigl, M., Disler, P., Jackel, W., van der Linden, S. and de Bie, R. (2004e). ICF core sets for low back pain. *Journal of Rehabilitation Medicine*, *44*(Supplement), 69–74.

Cieza, A., Schwarzkopf, S., Sigl, T., Stucki, G., Melvin, J., Stoll, T. and Walsh, N. (2004f). ICF core sets for osteoporosis. *Journal of Rehabilitation Medicine*, *44*(Supplement), 81–86.

Cieza, A., Geyh, S., Chatterji, S., Kostanjsek, N., Üstün, B. and Stucki, G. (2005). ICF linking rules: an update based on lessons learned. *Journal of Rehabilitation Medicine*, *37*(4), 212–218.

Cieza, A., Hilfiker, R., Boonen, A., Chatterji, S., Kostanjsek, N., Ustun, B. T. and Stucki, G. (2009). Items from patient-oriented instruments can be integrated into interval scales to operationalize categories of the International Classification of Functioning, Disability and Health. *Journal of Clinical Epidemiology*, *62*(9), 912–921.

Cieza, A., Kirchberger, I., Biering-Sorensen, F., Baumberger, M., Charlifue, S., Post, M. W. and Stucki, G. (2010). ICF core sets for individuals with spinal cord injury in the long-term context. *Spinal Cord*, *48*(4), 305–312.

Coenen, M., Cieza, A., Stamm, T. A., Amann, E., Kollerits, B. and Stucki, G. (2006). Validation of the International Classification of Functioning, Disability and Health (ICF) Core Set for rheumatoid arthritis from the patient perspective using focus groups. *Arthritis Research and Therapy*, *8*(4), R84.

Doyle, P. J., McNeil, M. R., Mikolic, J. M., Prieto, L., Hula, W. D., Lustig, A. P. and Elman, R. J. (2004). The Burden of Stroke Scale (BOSS) provides valid and reliable score estimates of functioning and well-being in stroke survivors with and without communication disorders. *Journal of Clinical Epidemiology*, *57*(10), 997–1007.

Dreinhofer, K., Stucki, G., Ewert, T., Huber, E., Ebenbichler, G., Gutenbrunner, C. and Cieza, A. (2004). ICF core sets for osteoarthritis. *Journal of Rehabilitation Medicine*, *44*(Supplement), 75–80.

Duncan, P. W., Lai, S. M., van Culin, V., Huang, L., Clausen, D. and Wallace, D. (1999). Development of a comprehensive assessment toolbox for stroke. *Clinical and Geriatric Medicine*, *15*(4), 885–915.

Eide, A. H., Jelsma, J., Loeb, M., Maart, S. and Toni, M. K. (2008). Exploring ICF components in a survey among Xhosa speakers in Eastern and Western Cape, South Africa. *Disability and Rehabilitation*, *30*(11), 819–829.

Engel, G. L. (1977). The need for a new medical model: a challenge for biomedicine. *Science*, *196*(4286), 129–136.

Fougeyrollas, P., Cloutier, R., Bergeron, H., Cote, J. and St Michel, G. (1998). *The Quebec Classification: Disability Creation Process*. Quebec: International Network on the Disability Creation Process; Canadian Society for the International Classification of Imparments, Disabilities and Handicaps.

Fugl-Meyer, A. R., Bränholm, I.-B. and Fugl-Meyer, K. S. (1991). Happiness and domain-specific life satisfaction in adult northern Swedes. *Clinical Rehabilitation*, *5*(1), 25–33.

Geyh, S., Cieza, A., Schouten, J., Dickson, H., Frommelt, P., Omar, Z. and Stucki, G. (2004). ICF core sets for stroke. *Journal of Rehabilitation Medicine*, *44*(Supplement), 135–141.

Geyh, S., Cieza, A., Kollerits, B., Grimby, G. and Stucki, G. (2007). Content comparison of health-related quality of life measures used in stroke based on the international classification of functioning, disability and health (ICF): a systematic review. *Quality of Life Research*, *16*(5), 833–851.

Gradinger, F., Cieza, A., Stucki, A., Michel, F., Bentley, A., Oksenberg, A. and Partinen, M. (2009). ICF core sets for persons with sleep disorders: results of the consensus process integrating evidence from preparatory studies. *Sleep Medicine*, *10*(Supplement 2), S12–S13.

Granger, C. V., Hamilton, B. B., Linacre, J. M., Heinemann, A. W. and Wright, B. D. (1993). Performance profiles of the functional independence measure. *American Journal of Physical Rehabilitation and Medicine*, *72*(2), 84–89.

Gutenbrunner, C., Ward, A. B. and Chamberlain, A. M. (2007). White book on Physical and Rehabilitation Medicine in Europe. *Journal of Rehabilitation Medicine*, *45*(Supplement), 6–47.

Heerkens, Y., Engels, J., Kuiper, C., Van der Gulden, J. and Oostendorp, R. (2004). The use of the ICF to describe work related factors influencing the health of employees. *Disability and Rehabilitation*, *26*(17), 1060–1066.

Hieblinger, R., Coenen, M., Stucki, G., Winkelmann, A. and Cieza, A. (2009). Validation of the International Classification of Functioning, Disability and Health Core Set for chronic widespread pain from the perspective of fibromyalgia patients. *Arthritis Research and Therapy*, *11*(3), R67.

Huber, J. G., Sillick, J. and Skarakis-Doyle, E. (2010). Personal perception and personal factors: incorporating health-related quality of life into the International Classification of Functioning, Disability and Health. *Disability and Rehabilitation*, *32*(23), 1955–1965.

Institute of Medicine, Pope, A. M. and Tarlov, A. R. (1991). *Disability in America: Toward a National Agenda for Prevention*. Washington, DC: National Academy Press.

Institute of Medicine, Brandt, E. N. and Pope, A. M. (1997). *Enabling America: Assessing the Role of Rehabilitation Science and Engineering*. Washington, DC: National Academy Press.

Institute of Medicine, Field, M. J. and Jette, A. M. (2007). *The Future of Disability in America*. Washington, DC: National Academy Press.

Jacob, R., Üstün, B., Madden, R. and Sykes, C. (2007). The WHO Family of International Classifications. *Bundesgesundheitsbl - Gesundheitsforsch – Gesundheitsschutz*, *50*, 924–931.

Kesselring, J., Coenen, M., Cieza, A., Thompson, A., Kostanjsek, N. and Stucki, G. (2008). Developing the ICF core sets for multiple sclerosis to specify functioning. *Multiple Sclerosis*, *14*(2), 252–254.

Khan, F. and Pallant, J.F. (2007a). Use of International Classification of Functioning, Disability and Health (ICF) to describe patient-reported disability in multiple sclerosis and identification of relevant environmental factors. *Journal of Rehabilitation Medicine*, *39*(1), 63–70.

Khan, F. and Pallant, J.F. (2007b). Use of the International Classification of Functioning, Disability and Health (ICF) to identify preliminary comprehensive and brief core sets for multiple sclerosis. *Disability and Rehabilitation*, *29*(3), 205–213.

Kielhofner, G. (2008). *Model of Human Occupation: Theory and Application*. Philadelphia, PA: Lippincott Williams and Wilkins.

Kirchberger, I., Coenen, M., Hierl, F. X., Dieterle, C., Seissler, J., Stucki, G. and Cieza, A. (2009). Validation of the International Classification of Functioning, Disability and Health (ICF) core set for diabetes mellitus from the patient perspective using focus groups. *Diabetes Medicine*, *26*(7), 700–707.

Kirchberger, I., Cieza, A., Biering-Sorensen, F., Baumberger, M., Charlifue, S., Post, M. W. and Stucki, G. (2010). ICF core sets for individuals with spinal cord injury in the early post-acute context. *Spinal Cord*, *48*(4), 297–304.

Kirchberger, I., Glaessel, A., Stucki, G. and Cieza, A. (2007). Validation of the comprehensive international classification of functioning, disability and health core set for rheumatoid arthritis: the perspective of physical therapists. *Physical Therapy*, *87*(4), 368–384.

Kostanjsek, N., Badley, E., De Kleijn, M. and Ustun, B. (2009). 'A man's reach should exceed his grasp' – In memory of Professor Philip Wood. *Disability and Rehabilitation*, *31*(17), 1389–1391.

Lemberg, I., Kirchberger, I., Stucki, G. and Cieza, A. (2010). The ICF core set for stroke from the perspective of physicians: a worldwide validation study using the Delphi technique. *European Journal of Physical and Rehabilitation Medicine*, *46*(3), 377–388.

Madden, R., Sykes, C. and Üstün, T. B. (2007). *World Health Organization Family of International Classifications: Definition, Scope and Purpose*. Geneva: WHO. http://www.who.int/classifications/en/FamilyDocument2007.pdf (accessed 30 August 2010).

Masala, C. and Petretto, D.R. (2008). From disablement to enablement: conceptual models of disability in the 20th century. *Disability and Rehabilitation*, *30*(17), 1233–1244.

McDougall, J., Wright, V. and Rosenbaum, P. (2010). The ICF model of functioning and disability: incorporating quality of life and human development. *Developmental Neurorehabilitation*, *13*(3), 204–211.

Nagi, S. Z. (1964). A Study in the Evaluation of Disability and Rehabilitation Potential: concepts, methods, and procedures. *American Journal of Public Health and the Nations Health*, *54*(9), 1568–1579.

Post, M. W. M., de Witte, L. P. and Schrijvers, A. J. P. (1999). Quality of life and the ICIDH: towards an integrated conceptual model for rehabilitation outcomes research. *Clinical Rehabilitation*, *13*, 5–15.

Post, M. W., de Witte, L. P., Reichrath, E., Verdonschot, M. M., Wijlhuizen, G. J. and Perenboom, R. J. (2008). Development and validation of IMPACT-S, an ICF-based questionnaire to measure activities and participation. *Journal of Rehabilitation Medicine*, *40*(8), 620–627.

Post, M. W., Kirchberger, I., Scheuringer, M., Wollaars, M. M. and Geyh, S. (2010). Outcome parameters in spinal cord injury research: a systematic review using the International Classification of Functioning, Disability and Health (ICF) as a reference. *Spinal Cord*, *48*(7), 522–528.

Raggi, A., Sirtori, A., Brunani, A., Liuzzi, A. and Leonardi, M. (2009). Use of the ICF to describe functioning and disability in obese patients. *Disability and Rehabilitation*, *31*(Supplement 1), S153–158.

Rauch, A., Cieza, A. and Stucki, G. (2008). How to apply the International Classification of Functioning, Disability and Health (ICF) for rehabilitation management in clinical practice. *European Journal of Physical and Rehabilitation Medicine*, *44*(3), 329–342.

Rauch, A., Kirchberger, I., Stucki, G. and Cieza, A. (2009). Validation of the Comprehensive ICF Core Set for obstructive pulmonary diseases from the perspective of physiotherapists. *Physiotherapy Research International*, *14*(4), 242–259.

Rauch, A., Bickenbach, J. E., Reinhardt, J. D., Geyh, S. and Stucki, G. (2010a). The utility of the ICF to identify and evaluate problems and needs in participation in spinal cord injury rehabilitation. *Topics in Spinal Cord Injury Rehabilitation*, *15*(4), 72–86.

Rauch, A., Escorpizo, R., Riddle, D. L., Eriks-Hoogland, I., Stucki, G. and Cieza, A. (2010b). Using a case report of a patient with spinal cord injury to illustrate the application of the international classification of functioning, disability and health during multidisciplinary patient management. *Physical Therapy*, *90*(7), 1039–1052.

Roe, C., Sveen, U., Cieza, A., Geyh, S. and Bautz-Holter, E. (2009). Validation of the Brief ICF core set for low back pain from the Norwegian perspective. *European Journal of Physical and Rehabilitation Medicine*, *45*(3), 403–414.

Ruof, J., Cieza, A., Wolff, B., Angst, F., Ergeletzis, D., Omar, Z. and Stucki, G. (2004). ICF core sets for diabetes mellitus. *Journal of Rehabilitation Medicine*, *44*(Supplement), 100–106.

Salter, K., Jutai, J. W., Teasell, R., Foley, N. C. and Bitensky, J. (2005a). Issues for selection of outcome measures in stroke rehabilitation: ICF Body Functions. *Disability and Rehabilitation*, *27*(4), 191–207.

Salter, K., Jutai, J. W., Teasell, R., Foley, N. C., Bitensky, J. and Bayley, M. (2005b). Issues for selection of outcome measures in stroke rehabilitation: ICF activity. *Disability and Rehabilitation*, *27*(6), 315–340.

Salter, K., Jutai, J. W., Teasell, R., Foley, N. C., Bitensky, J. and Bayley, M. (2005c). Issues for selection of outcome measures in stroke rehabilitation: ICF Participation. *Disability and Rehabilitation*, *27*(9), 507–528.

Starrost, K., Geyh, S., Trautwein, A., Grunow, J., Ceballos-Baumann, A., Prosiegel, M. and Cieza, A. (2008). Interrater reliability of the extended ICF core set for stroke applied by physical therapists. *Physical Therapy*, *88*(7), 841–851.

Steiner, W. A., Ryser, L., Huber, E., Uebelhart, D., Aeschlimann, A. and Stucki, G. (2002). Use of the ICF model as a clinical problem-solving tool in physical therapy and rehabilitation medicine. *Physical Therapy*, *82*(11), 1098–1107.

Stephens, D. and Kerr, P. (2000). Auditory disablements: an update. *Audiology*, *39*(6), 322–332.

Stucki, G., Cieza, A., Ewert, T., Kostanjsek, N., Chatterji, S. and Ustun, T. (2002). Application of the International Classification of Functioning, Disability and Health (ICF) in clinical practice. *Disability and Rehabilitation*, *24*(5), 281–282.

Stucki, G., Ewert, T. and Cieza, A. (2003). Value and application of the ICF in rehabilitation medicine. *Disability and Rehabilitation*, *25*(11–12), 628–634.

Stucki, A., Daansen, P., Fuessl, M., Cieza, A., Huber, E., Atkinson, R. and Ruof, J. (2004a). ICF core sets for obesity. *Journal of Rehabilitation Medicine*, *44*(Supplement), 107–113.

Stucki, A., Stoll, T., Cieza, A., Weigl, M., Giardini, A., Wever, D. and Stucki, G. (2004b). ICF core sets for obstructive pulmonary diseases. *Journal of Rehabilitation Medicine*, *44*(Supplement), 114–120.

Stucki, G., Cieza, A., Geyh, S., Battistella, L., Lloyd, J., Symmons, D. and Schouten, J. (2004c). ICF core sets for rheumatoid arthritis. *Journal of Rehabilitation Medicine*, *44*(Supplement), 87–93.

Swiss Paraplegic Research. (2007). *Implementation of the International Classification of Functioning, Disability and Health (ICF) in rehabilitation practice*. Nottwil: Swiss Paraplegic Research. www.icf-casestudies.org (accessed 5 March 2012).

Taylor, W. J., Mease, P. J., Adebajo, A., Nash, P. J., Feletar, M. and Gladman, D. D. (2010). Effect of psoriatic arthritis according to the affected categories of the International Classification of Functioning, Disability and Health. *Journal of Rheumatology*, *37*(9), 1885–1891.

Tschiesner, U., Cieza, A., Rogers, S. N., Piccirillo, J., Funk, G., Stucki, G. and Berghaus, A. (2007). Developing core sets for patients with head and neck cancer based on the International Classification of Functioning, Disability and Health (ICF). *European Archives of Otorhinolaryngology*, *264*(10), 1215–1222.

Tschiesner, U. M., Chen, A., Funk, G., Yueh, B. and Rogers, S. N. (2009). Shortfalls in international, multidisciplinary outcome data collection following head and neck cancer: does the ICF Core Set for HNC provide a common solution? *Oral Oncology*, *45*(10), 849–855.

Tschiesner, U., Rogers, S., Dietz, A., Yueh, B. and Cieza, A. (2010). Development of ICF core sets for head and neck cancer. *Head Neck*, *32*(2), 210–220.

Ueda, S. and Okawa, Y. (2003). The subjective dimension of functioning and disability: what is it and what is it for? *Disability and Rehabilitation*, *25*(11–12), 596–601.

Uhlig, T., Lillemo, S., Moe, R. H., Stamm, T., Cieza, A., Boonen, A. and Stucki, G. (2007). Reliability of the ICF core set for rheumatoid arthritis. *Annals of the Rheumatic Diseases*, *66*(8), 1078–1084.

Uhlig, T., Moe, R., Reinsberg, S., Kvien, T. K., Cieza, A. and Stucki, G. (2009). Responsiveness of the International Classification of Functioning, Disability and Health (ICF) core set for rheumatoid arthritis. *Annals of the Rheumatic Diseases*, *68*(6), 879–884.

Union of the Physically Impaired Against Segregation (UPIAS). (1975). *Fundemental Principles of Disability*. London: UPIAS. http://www.leeds.ac.uk/disability-studies/archiveuk/UPIAS/fundamental%20principles.pdf (accessed on 5 December 2011).

Ustun, T. B., Cooper, J. E., van Duuren-Kristen, S., Kennedy, C., Hendershot, G. and Sartorius, N. (1995). Revision of the ICIDH: mental health aspects. *WHO/MNH Disability Working Group. Disability and Rehabilitation*, *17*(3–4), 202–209.

Ustun, T. B., Chatterji, S., Bickenbach, J., Kostanjsek, N. and Schneider, M. (2003). The International Classification of Functioning, Disability and Health: a new tool for understanding disability and health. *Disability and Rehabilitation*, 25(11–12), 565–571.

Ustun, B., Chatterji, S. and Kostanjsek, N. (2004). Comments from WHO for the Journal of Rehabilitation Medicine Special Supplement on ICF core sets. *Journal of Rehabilitation Medicine*, 44(Supplement), 7–8.

van der Zee, C. H., Priesterbach, A. R., van der Dussen, L., Kap, A., Schepers, V. P. M., Visser-Meily, J. M. A. and Post, M. W. M. (2010). Reproducibility of three self-report participation measures: the ICF measure of participation and activities screener, the participation scale and the utrecht scale for evaluation of rehabilitation-participation. *Journal of Rehabilitation Medicine*, 42(8), 752–757.

Vieta, E., Cieza, A., Stucki, G., Chatterji, S., Nieto, M., Sanchez-Moreno, J. and Ayuso-Mateos, J. L. (2007). Developing core sets for persons with bipolar disorder based on the International Classification of Functioning, Disability and Health. *Bipolar Disorders*, 9(1–2), 16–24.

Viol, M., Grotkamp, S., van Treeck, B., Nuchtern, E., Hagen, T., Manegold, B. and Seger, W. (2006). Personal contextual factors, part I (in German). *Gesundheitswesen*, 68(12), 747–759.

Whiteneck, G. (2005). Conceptual models of disability: past, present, and future. In M. J. Field, A. M. Jette and L. Martin (Editors). *Disability in America. A New Look*. I. Washington: National Academies Press, pp. 50–66.

Whiteneck, G. G. (2010). Issues affecting the selection of participation measurement in outcomes research and clinical trials. *Archives of Physical Medicine and Rehabilitation*, 91(9 Supplement), S54–59.

Whiteneck, G. and Dijkers, M. P. (2009). Difficult to measure constructs: conceptual and methodological issues concerning participation and environmental factors. *Archives of Physical Medicine and Rehabilitation*, 90(11 Supplement), S22–35.

World Health Organization. (1980). *International Classification of Impairments, Disabilities and Handicaps*. Geneva: WHO.

World Health Organization. (1992). *International Statistical Classification of Diseases and Related Health Problems (10th revision)*. Geneva: WHO.

World Health Organization. (2000). *World Health Organisation Disability Assessment Schedule (WHODASII). Training Manual: A Guide to Administration*. Geneva: WHO.

World Health Organization. (2001). *International Classification of Functioning, Disability and Health: ICF*. Geneva: WHO.

World Health Organization. (2002). *Towards a Common Language for Functioning, Disability and Health: ICF*. Geneva: World Health Organization.

World Health Organization. (2007). *ICF-CY. International Classification of Functioning, Disability and Health. Children and Youth Version*. Geneva: WHO.

Xie, F., Lo, N. N., Lee, H. P., Cieza, A. and Li, S. C. (2007). Validation of the Comprehensive ICF Core Set for Osteoarthritis (OA) in patients with knee OA: a Singaporean perspective. *Journal of Rheumatology*, 34(11), 2301–2307.

Chapter 3

An interprofessional approach to rehabilitation

Sarah G. Dean[1] *and Claire Ballinger*[2]

[1] *Senior Lecturer in Health Services Research, University of Exeter Medical School, United Kingdom;* [2] *Deputy Director/Senior Qualitative Health Research Fellow, National Institute for Health Research (NIHR) Research Design Service South Central, University of Southampton, United Kingdom*

3.1 Introduction and setting the scene

Clinical rehabilitation teams have been in existence since the early 1900s when the first schools of physical therapy were opened and army hospitals were established to deal with the challenges presented by wounded personnel during the two world wars (Dillingham, 2002). Given the complexity of problems faced by these and other casualties it made sense to bring together people from different professional and disciplinary backgrounds. Throughout the intervening decades rehabilitation teams have varied in their structure, membership and procedures. To continue with the military example, Selly Oak Hospital, the Royal Centre of Defence Medicine in Birmingham, has become the place where British casualties from the war in Afghanistan are sent. Many of these service personnel have complex injuries including multiple limb loss; the Selly Oak teams provide acute care and the early stages of rehabilitation, with longer-term rehabilitation being undertaken at the Defence Medical Rehabilitation Centre at Headley Court. The role of the rehabilitation teams for these complex cases was depicted in the award-winning BBC documentary called 'Wounded' made in 2009, as they followed the rehabilitation of several soldiers with multiple limb amputation. Outcomes for British combat amputees indicate that more individuals are surviving complex and severe injuries than previously, rehabilitation provides significant benefit regarding self-reported physical functioning and the majority successfully return to military work (Dharm-Datta et al., 2011).

So much has been recorded about the importance of rehabilitation teams and of working together as a team and in this chapter we aim to show that there are different ways of viewing roles within a team. Our purpose in doing this is to encourage

Interprofessional Rehabilitation: A Person-Centred Approach, First Edition.
Edited by Sarah G. Dean, Richard J. Siegert and William J. Taylor.
© 2012 John Wiley & Sons, Ltd. Published 2012 by John Wiley & Sons, Ltd.

reflection to help team members consider how their skills, roles and attributes can be best configured to provide the best outcome for the service user.

In this chapter we will explore the issue of professional and disciplinary identity and how all stakeholders in the rehabilitation process, including the service user, view their contributions to the overall endeavour. We start by reviewing key issues surrounding terminology employed in rehabilitation practice and go on to consider some of the defining features of good team work, both within rehabilitation and more widely from fields of health and management, in order to suggest characteristics against which the performance of rehabilitation teams might be evaluated. We also look at different types of membership and roles within the team, the processes of team working and in particular team meetings and collaborative practice. We also take into account the requirements for effective interprofessional assessment and consider how the domains of education, practice and research influence interprofessional rehabilitation.

Throughout this chapter, we draw on a number of different practice examples, in particular from the field of falls prevention for and with older people, a specialist area requiring the skills and expertise from many rehabilitation professionals, in addition to participation from older adults themselves.

3.2 Terminology and interprofessional working within rehabilitation

One issue that has the potential to cause great confusion within rehabilitation is that of the language routinely used within practice. Terms such as 'multidisciplinary' and 'interprofessional' are often used to describe a team approach in practice without much thought to which term is best or most appropriate to use. We argue that there are subtle differences in meaning and that careful consideration of the language used to describe the delivery of rehabilitation is important. Such consideration can be more widely reflective of a thoughtful and jointly negotiated approach to service provision, which in turn may also result in a positive impact on the health outcomes obtained from the service.

Within the context of teamwork the use of the prefixes 'inter' or 'multi' to go with the words 'disciplinary' or 'professional' result in some of the most interchangeably used terms within rehabilitation. For example, these terms may mean the team is made up of people representing very different professions or disciplines. Alternatively, a multidisciplinary team may comprise people from the same profession but who represent different specialist disciplines within that profession, for example, in the care of a child with spina bifida the medical team is likely to include a paediatrician, urologist, orthopaedic surgeon, neurosurgeon and rehabilitation physician. Although often dismissed as 'mere semantics', the choice of terminology is worthy of some deliberation as, in addition to describing or reflecting entities and actions, language also has the potential to construct social realities (Potter, 1996). For example, the language that has been used to describe services to prevent falls and their clients, has been discussed by Yardley and others. These authors suggest that the term 'faller' has a potentially undesirable effect, resulting in reduced uptake of such services (Yardley et al., 2007; see also Ballinger and Payne, 2002). Similarly, Holliday and colleagues have demonstrated how a term such as 'goal' can be adopted relatively easily by healthcare staff, but be interpreted in a variety of different ways by service users. The term 'goal' is not always regarded positively and may even result in a detrimental effect on the service user (Holliday et al., 2007; Van de Weyer et al., 2010) (see also Chapter 4 for more about the use of goals in rehabilitation).

In contemplating the terms 'discipline' and 'profession', the personal perspective of one of the authors of this chapter, Sarah, is useful in thinking about the use of different terms. Sarah has a dual background and education in health psychology and physiotherapy. This presents interesting challenges in underlying philosophy, for example, when asked to introduce herself to new colleagues. Health psychology is considered an academic discipline, or deriving from a body of knowledge that has emerged from the wider field of study, psychology. As a discipline, it has concentrated on academic research and theoretical development (British Psychological Society, www.bps.org.uk) but more recently has focused on the application of health psychology to practice, with the Health Professions Council's psychologist register opening in 2009 (http://www.hpc-uk.org/). In contrast, physiotherapy has developed as a practising profession with professional autonomy legally established in 1978 (Chartered Society of Physiotherapy, www.csp.org.uk). The physiotherapy profession is characterized by practice and the clinical application of its treatment approaches; theory has been developed from this clinical expertise and only relatively recently has there been a strong push for physiotherapists to engage with research and to explore scientifically whether physiotherapy interventions are effective or not (Barnard and Wiles, 2001; Herbert et al., 2001).

The key issue here is that neither 'discipline' nor 'profession' are intrinsically more worthy, appropriate or better, but rather that they each are more meaningful within different contexts. As a lecturer working within a university, for example, Sarah's colleagues throughout the institution will be more familiar with the notion of academic disciplines as a means of distinguishing activity and outputs, such as papers and conference presentations. Her identity as a psychologist will have more salience and credibility, deriving from psychology's extensive tradition of research and scholarly activity. However, within the context of a practice-based setting, such as a clinical service, there is likely to be more understanding about Sarah's alternative identity as a physiotherapist, a profession with which more service providers and users will be familiar, with greater public visibility, and which many will have encountered. Within such a service setting, the delivery of applied interventions will be prioritized, and often more highly valued than more cerebral academic endeavours. We will return to this example a little later on in the chapter, when we examine the tensions that can arise when determining the boundaries of professional practice for someone who works in an interprofessional setting.

Often overlooked in relation to the choice of terminology in rehabilitation teamwork are the people who may not be explicitly regarded as members of the team. For example, unqualified service providers, such as porters, reception staff or cleaners, may not be seen as part of the team and yet they can be crucial to the smooth operation of a service. Other examples of unacknowledged members of the team are the service users, such as the person who has survived a stroke and their families or carers. The term 'professional' suggests that only people with a recognized professional education, such as those who are eligible for registration with the Health Professions Council in the UK, can be included within the team. Similarly, the notion of 'discipline' implies that the knowledge or expertise is located with those from within the discipline, which can also be perceived as exclusive. Within the context of falls prevention, one of the ways in which this problem has been addressed is to describe the team in terms of health or social care staff, but to also identify that the team works in collaboration with other people. Thus, there may be active participation of services users, their families and carers within the team (see for example: the Active Living Falls Prevention and Functional Ability programme in Wigan, http://www.getactivewiganandleigh.co.uk/active-living-programmes/active-later-life/).

Although we have discussed the use of both 'profession(al)' and 'discipline(ary)' in relation to descriptions of rehabilitation teamwork, we would argue that of greater importance is the choice of a prefix from 'inter', 'multi' or 'trans' (disciplinary/professional), and we next want to describe and distinguish between these, in order to encourage a clearer focus on the nature and scope of teamwork.

Perhaps the term used most frequently to describe groups of healthcare staff who work together in a rehabilitation context is 'multidisciplinary'. Derick Wade, a prominent UK rehabilitation physician, has consistently used this term in describing rehabilitation practice (e.g. Wade, 2000). In a widely cited paper, Wade and de Jong outline the structure of a rehabilitation service in the following terms: '...a multidisciplinary team of people who: work together towards common goals for each patient; involve and educate the patient and family; have relevant knowledge and skills; can resolve most of the common problems faced by their patients' (Wade and de Jong, 2000, p. 1386).

The ideal of joint working is described within this framework but we argue that the focus may still be on the 'many parts' or individual specialist roles coming together to contribute to the rehabilitation package of care. This raises the concern that it will result in prioritization of personal professional culture, practices and ethos over the collective team effort and this is likely to be to the detriment of the service user. Within such a multidisciplinary approach each team member might potentially carry out their own assessment and formulate their own treatment plan, even though they are ostensibly committed to the joint aim of optimizing function and enhancing participation of the patient. This is potentially confusing for service users and families, and can lead to disjointed and patchy service provision. In a worst case scenario there might be a guarding of professional skills and interventions, characterized by unwritten rules about who does what, which treatment approaches 'belong' to which profession and what, if any, degree of transfer of skills and activities is allowed across the professions. In this scenario physiotherapists, for example, may not believe it is appropriate for nurses to loan walking aids such as crutches, or perhaps that it is appropriate for a nurse to use a walking aid such as a zimmer frame to help someone to reach the toilet but not appropriate for the nurse to teach a patient user how to use a pair of crutches on the stairs before they are discharged home. Boundaries between roles and remits within a multidisciplinary team might be rigid or relatively flexible, but characteristically each profession retains its autonomy and values. This could result in retention of professional boundaries remaining a higher priority than provision of a responsive and flexible service in which service user needs are foremost. Consequently there may be little incentive to alter the existing structures that relate to the participating health professions, and it becomes unlikely that others will share, cover or take over another's role. So autonomy for each discipline remains, and changes in structure or theoretical approach are less likely to occur (Gibbons et al., 1994). This tension, between professional autonomy and teamwork, can be addressed constructively. The following case study illustrates this point within the context of a falls clinic, where the teamwork resulted in beneficial health outcomes for a service user.

Case study

Mrs Violet Greenwood, aged 86, was referred to her local falls prevention clinic by her general practitioner (GP), following a fall that had resulted in severe bruising. On assessment it was revealed that Mrs Greenwood had been having a number of falls, but it was only after the recent fall that she had gone to see her GP. The assessment team included physiotherapists, occupational therapists, nurses and a geriatrician. They identified a number of factors that were likely to be contributing to Mrs Greenwood's situation. These factors included impairments of body structures and function: lower limb muscle weakness, poor balance, painful thumb joints and swollen feet. Mrs Greenwood was also limited in some of her activities of daily living, such as getting up and down from a chair, walking, gripping and holding items. The assessment team also noted a number of environmental factors that were likely to be making the situation even more difficult for Mrs Greenwood: a walking stick that was the wrong height and had no ferrule; large slippers with a slit at their front (Mrs Greenwood preferred to wear these because of her swollen feet). All these factors resulted in Mrs Greenwood being restricted in her ability to participate in living independently although her priority was to continue to prepare simple meals and hot drinks for herself.

Individual members of the team provided a number of solutions. For example, the physiotherapist suggested some simple home exercises to improve leg muscle strength and balance and to decrease the swelling in her feet as well as providing a correctly sized walking stick with a new ferrule. The occupational therapist provided adapted kitchen equipment including a kettle tipper, and arranged for Mrs Greenwood to have her feet correctly fitted with comfortable but supportive shoes. The geriatrician reviewed medication with particular attention to polypharmacy (multiple prescriptions) that might be interacting or causing balance problems. However, the team identified some critical principles that needed to underpin service provision with Mrs Greenwood: consistency and reinforcement. Thus, the occupational therapist helped support the exercise programme by discussing with Mrs Greenwood how she might remember to carry it out, and reinforced the need for using the walking stick indoors. The physiotherapist encouraged Mrs Greenwood to wear her new shoes, and demonstrated how they provided more support. She also discussed where the exercises might be carried out during the daily routine, for example, toe raises while standing at the sink prior to making tea. With Mrs Greenwood's consent, both therapists invited Mrs Greenwood's daughter to attend several early treatment sessions to demonstrate different elements of the intervention, and to show the daughter how Mrs Greenwood responded very positively to consistent encouragement. A community nurse who did a follow-up visit 4 weeks later found that Mrs Greenwood was more confident about her mobility, was continuing to live independently, had not reported any further falls and was able to make them both a cup of tea.

The professionals in the team described in Mrs Greenwood's case were still operating within their traditional roles but had agreed some joint and underpinning approaches to the various interventions required by Mrs Greenwood, so they were going some way towards working interprofessionally. Generally however, the prefix 'inter' (as in interprofessional or interdisciplinary) suggests more potential overlap in roles, with boundaries being blurred or relaxed. This might be a consequence of a team having been together for some time, secure in their professional skills and knowledge, but having a more sophisticated understanding of team members' strengths, preferences and styles. As an example, the second author of this chapter, Claire, joined a relatively new community learning disability team in which interventions were initially offered according to professional demarcation (so the physiotherapist and speech and language therapist jointly offered a communications and exercise class). As the team matured and became more confident and trusting, creative solutions to client-oriented problems evolved that were less reflective of professional domains. Latterly the team chartered a canal boat for clients, this provided respite care for families but also a variety of opportunities for learning through practice (see Chapter 6 for more about this). The clients practised food preparation skills, the trip facilitated community engagement through stopping at public houses along the canal waterways for an evening drink and provided clients with the opportunity to learn about a new leisure activity. Canal locks, getting on and off of the boat, and standing on the deck and in the interior offered strength, transfer and balance challenges, and steering the canal boat provided a popular opportunity to be in control and empowered. This move to an interprofessional framework can signify a more holistic way of working, characterized by sharing and knowledge transfer between team members. This facilitates effective teamwork and enables the team to create its own momentum and ethos, resulting in a whole that is greater than the sum of its parts, a point that we will return to later in this chapter.

Another relatively new approach to rehabilitation teamwork is 'transdisciplinary' practice. King et al. (2005) describe transdisciplinary rehabilitation teams as promoting cross-treatment with the service user centrally involved, sharing responsibilities and a blurring of roles. Advantages include valuing of information transfer, lack of any specific role dominance and expansion of professional expertise, resulting in more effective provision. One of the key mechanisms for promoting transdisciplinary working is joint training or education. Browner and Bessire (2004) provide an example of how this was achieved, through the contribution of senior staff from all rehabilitation professions, within the context of the development of basic competency education modules for staff working with brain and spinal cord injured people. The modules were delivered to 95 of the 110 staff members working within a rehabilitation facility over a 4-day 'Competency Fair'. Positive outcomes included greater appreciation of each others' roles, empowerment to share roles, greater crossover of duties, a better understanding of transdisciplinary care, improvements in patient care and increase in knowledge. Just as we mentioned in the example given in the section about interdisciplinary approaches, the move to a transdisciplinary culture may take some time. Various authors have investigated what might be needed for this development to occur, and King et al. discuss Walker and Avant's (1995) five premises that are likely to be required before it is possible to apply this approach to rehabilitation: (1) role extension; (2) role enrichments; (3) role expansion; (4) role release, and (5) role support (King et al., 2005). We have used the example of working with patients, who have chronic low back pain and are attending a chronic pain clinic, to suggest ways in which these conditions might be achieved in rehabilitation (see Table 3.1). In addition, an effective transdisciplinary team can be characterized by stability of staff (i.e. low turnover) and an underpinning philosophy of co-operation and collaboration as opposed to individual (professional) achievement.

The different terms that are frequently encountered when describing the overall structure of a rehabilitation team reveal how some subtle differences in terminology can have the potential to influence how well a team might work. We go on to discuss some of the characteristics that enable a team to work well together, and some of the common problems that can occur within teams.

3.3   Characteristics of good teamwork

Perhaps one of the first introductions to the notion of teamwork to which we are exposed as children is during school physical education. Some will have had experience of playing for the year or school team – perhaps rounders, football or netball. Sporting teams have their own distinct roles and rules, but in considering the characteristics of a good rehabilitation team, reflection on successful sports team can prove illuminating. Similarly within commerce, successful businesses are often the product of a close cohesive team, sharing similar aspirations, loyalties and ethos. So as trainee health professionals, we tend to be reasonably familiar with the idea of teams.

Teams that work well and teams that work less well

When reflecting on flourishing teams, there is often a tendency to attribute success to personal characteristics of team members, such as a strong leader, loyal members and individuals with creativity or confidence. However, the organisational and environmental context within which a team operates, although receiving less attention, is as important as any individual traits in facilitating effective performance. These contextual factors are recognized within theory about team performance and these contextual factors are also important for influencing how performance can be maintained over time. Drinka and Clark (2000) for example, identify factors at three different levels that have an impact on healthcare team performance. At the first level are both personal factors (such as communications skills, leadership style and maturity) and professional factors (these include expertise, dedication to an ideal and knowledge of roles of others). At the second level intra-team issues relate to structure, for example formal leadership, norms and physical placement and process issues relate to goal setting, building trust and managing conflict. At the third level organizational issues are both internal, such as team philosophy, resource allocation and rigid or flexible

Table 3.1   Potential facilitators for transdisciplinary working in a chronic pain team: examples based on Walker and Avant's (1995) five premises and King et al.'s (2005) discussion points.

Premise	Potential facilitators
Role extension	• Being secure in one's own professional identity yet still extending knowledge and skills through training and continuing professional development • Undertaking activities that stretch the boundaries of what is considered 'usual practice' within the context of the professional role. For example, musculoskeletal physiotherapists training in Western acupuncture for use as a complementary intervention for pain relief • Being aware of how one's own professional contribution to patient care is complemented by the contributions from other professions. For example, strategies to decrease a patient's level of stress (and hence low back pain experience) could be a combination of muscle relaxation exercises taught by a physiotherapist and stress management techniques led by a psychologist
Role enrichments	• Further awareness and knowledge of other professions and their treatment approaches, for example, pacing (occupational therapists) and cognitive–behavioural therapy (psychologists) and their ways of working (assessment procedures, treatment planning etc) • Using this knowledge to create collective working practices and implement integrated approaches to treatment (e.g. shared assessment forms or goal planning documentation) • Team building days with a focus on the team dynamics and communication skills within the team
Role expansion	• Sharing and disseminating knowledge about your own profession to others. For example, a physiotherapist might teach the other professionals in the team about the principles of good posture when sitting at the computer to reduce neck and low back pain; the psychologist may offer an in-service team training session about how the team can use cognitive–behavioural approaches for the management of patients with chronic low back pain
Role release	• Joint working with other professions with some blurring of traditional boundaries. For example, all professions work using the principles of cognitive–behavioural approaches to pain management; all clinic staff ensure patients have appropriate seating and postural support during assessment and follow-up interviews • Agreed work on special projects for the whole team. For example, the implementation of a common assessment form or outcome measure that all professions will use
Role support	• Guidance, encouragement and feedback to team members who have adopted a joint practice. For example, a psychologist noticing and giving positive feedback to a physiotherapist who has taken time to address fear of movement when teaching a patient to perform exercises for managing low back pain • Encouragement and support of best practice for timely pain management to staff working in other settings of the same hospital

rules, and external issues, for example national policy and funding. We can learn from industrial and organizational psychology literature (for example Guzzo and Shea, 1992) about some established variables upon which effective teamwork relies and apply this to interprofessional rehabilitation.

- Task interdependence: the extent to which team members must interact to achieve a goal. In the earlier case study involving Mrs Greenwood this would mean all team members using the principles of 'consistency and reinforcement'.
- Outcome interdependence: the degree to which responsibility for the outcome and any consequences are shared within the team, regardless of the success or otherwise of these outcomes. In Mrs Greenwood's case this would mean whether or not she went on to have another fall, or moved into residential care.
- Potency or team self-efficacy: the belief that the team has the necessary skills, attributes and resources to achieve the desired goals. In the example the team needs to be confident that they have effective communication procedures and sufficient resources in order to be consistent in what and how they are asking Mrs Greenwood to undertake rehabilitation activities, and that the same messages are being reinforced.

(Adapted from Guzzo and Shea, 1992)

These authors describe 'resources' as 'environmental supports', similar to the organizational factors identified by Drinka and Clark (2000), and it is clear that the environmental context can have an impact on team performance. One of the most obvious environmental contextual factors that has an impact on the capacity of a team to reflect on, appraise and evaluate its own performance is time. When time to work with patients is limited there is likely to be a tendency for the team to focus solely on patient needs as perceived at that moment and in the immediate context that person is in. This is likely to lead to task-orientated care and fewer team interactions, with these tasks often mistakenly described as goals (see Chapter 4 for more detail on goals). If we take the example of an older patient who has experienced a fall, the 'goal' might be to work towards 'independent mobility', an activity which if done safely and successfully might be a regarded as 'goal' achieved, but probably only by one professional group (for example, physiotherapists or occupational therapists). However, a closer analysis of the situation reveals that the important goal is really about being able to perform kitchen activities of daily living after they have been discharged home, in particular being able to make a cup of tea. Ward-based physiotherapists and occupational therapists therefore work with the patient to build strength and promote balance, they rehearse kitchen-based activities with support, nurses encourage and reinforce use to increase confidence; family members learn when to help and when to stand back; and community-based therapists check how the home kitchen layout supports or hinders easy completion of key kitchen tasks. Although the original goal identified by the time-pressed team was not wrong, the original goal of 'independent mobility' was not a sufficiently detailed analysis, and lacked collaboration of input or involvement of the patient to guide the whole team.

Sometimes when there is limited time the opposite problem will occur, so that instead of the focus being on the individual activities, the team will announce a big 'goal', for example, to discharge the patient home. Again this might be an important aim for all concerned and so worthy of pursuit. However, there may only be an implicit understanding of this type of goal as it has not been fully articulated among the team members, and nor is there any consensus about how it is to be achieved and who will be contributing which element. It is also possible that both these events take place within the time-pressed team so an implicit broad goal of discharge home co-exists with the generation of a range of isolated tasks. These tasks may be devoid of context and lack coherence despite the fact that each professional thinks they will be needed.

All this suggests that effective teamwork stems from a balance of understanding and by accurately describing patient circumstances, and carrying out the necessary actions required to address these circumstances. This requires the skill to analyse the often complex needs of the service user and their family in their specific context. Using the example of referral following a fall, issues that require careful assessment will include personal factors, such as coping with disability or loss, confidence, self-efficacy and other psychosocial factors. In addition the assessment may also need to consider the perhaps more obvious physical needs a person has. This will also include environmental factors such as the availability of community resources or residential care, the need for a home environment that is safe and provides cues to activity, maybe through the use of telecare. In occupational therapy one of the most widely used models of practice is the Canadian Model of Occupational Performance (Canadian Association of Occupational Therapists, 1997) and its latest iteration includes the addition of engagement (Townsend and Polatajko 2007). From this model the Canadian Occupational Performance Measure (Baptiste et al., 2005) has been developed to guide therapists in their assessment process, so that the person, their 'occupations' or activities in relation to self-care, leisure and productivity, and the environment are all taken into account. Although this outcome measure is derived from an occupational therapy model of practice, it has been used within interdisciplinary rehabilitation research to provide a comprehensive evaluation of the effectiveness of a rehabilitation intervention (e.g. Esnouf et al., 2010).

Other contextual factors that can have an impact on the success of interprofessional teams are the systems that are in place and the availability of processes such as assessments, key worker systems and team meetings. Such processes can facilitate the co-ordination and delivery of packages of rehabilitation from a variety of team members who are aiming to address complex needs. For instance, an older patient who has had a hip fracture following a fall wants to go home and a key issue for her is the preservation of her autonomy. In order to support her desire for autonomy (and to help her test out its practicality) the physiotherapist and occupational therapist may assist in improving her walking and they may help to modify her home and routines to promote safety and independence. The nursing staff provide encouragement and help to motivate her while in hospital to maintain her activities of daily living and her physician provides support and monitoring through evaluating the fracture healing process. The social worker provides information about support systems and works with key family members over the right for older people to take risks and the family's ability to assist in an unobtrusive monitoring process. Simultaneously, the social worker may be involved in working with the patient on modifying unrealistic expectations about speed and extent of recovery. Rather than identifying tasks, the team, in this scenario, seeks to think about the issues confronting the person before moving on to identify the tasks that relate to working with those issues.

The use of systems and processes that underpin provision of support for complex needs can enable team members to contextualize and link their very different modes of intervention. It will also help them to identify the relationships between the different issues and concerns that patients have to manage. This assists in the provision of integrative care and also enables team members to identify and discuss differences in interpretation of those issues. In the above scenario a discussion might be warranted concerning identification of risk, and whether there is consensus about an acceptable level of risk. Similarly, it would be useful to share and compare views about when each team member would intervene and why. Shared reflection creates learning opportunities for the interprofessional rehabilitation team. In this example it might permit exploration of members' different ways of defining risk and their emotional responses to the issue of risk assessment, including how this affects older people and how this has implications for service provision.

To provide a further understanding of the skills and expertise of members of the rehabilitation team, organizational factors such as staff availability, rehabilitation resources and networks of communication with other agencies are also required. The development of systematic, reflective and service-user focused practice is not easy, and requires attention to team activities such as discussion, goal setting and decision making. What is of some concern is that rehabilitation professionals may lack training in, and detailed knowledge of, teamwork and group processes. In order to maximize the effectiveness of teamwork, team members need to be able to contribute to a facilitative team process. They need to be able to analyse their contribution to the process as well as evaluate the overall process itself. In addition to this, good teamwork requires solid knowledge about others' work and roles, as well as the ability to discuss and convey the key dimensions of one's own role.

Models of successful teamwork in other health settings can be helpful in identifying characteristics to which interprofessional rehabilitation teams might aspire. Boon et al. (2004) for example, describe a conceptual framework for evaluating different types of team practices in the provision of healthcare, focusing on four dimensions: philosophy, structure, process and outcomes. They illustrate how these four dimensions operate along a continuum for different varieties of healthcare teams and these can be characterized according to their degree of integration. By way of example, they suggest that a service user with acute myocardial infarction will benefit most from a team able to respond rapidly. In this situation it is likely that the team philosophy will be very biomedically based and orientated towards saving life, the team structure will comprise highly independent practitioners, team processes relatively rigid and rehearsed, with outcomes measured in terms of mortality. Conversely, a service user with long-term, complex needs (such as an older person experiencing frequent falls living in the community) is likely to benefit from a rehabilitation team that works in a more integrated fashion. Here, the team philosophy will be about maximizing the capabilities of the individual, team structures and processes will be less rigid, and outcomes are likely to be measured in terms of improving quality of life through reducing falls, improving confidence and/or enhancing mobility (or at least minimizing any deterioration in quality of life). So in preference to saying that a fully integrated team is always the ideal, Boon et al. (2004) rather suggest that this framework can help facilitate service users and providers to decide which model suits their needs best.

In another example of designing successful teamwork Wake-Dyster (2001) describes a project undertaken in paediatric services to explain the implementation of teamwork in a number of different child health teams, including a rehabilitation service. Success was attributed to a number of key features including the following:

- A 'team vision' and 'strong commitment to teamwork and patient care improvements' that were not just focused on clinical goals but provided a sense of accountability within the team for achieving results.
- Processes to guide team development including leaders' awareness and 'acceptance of "where staff are at"'.
- Building of 'leadership capacity' and 'cross-team learning' with acknowledgement of the need for flexibility.
- Including opportunities for 'encouragement and to experience success'.
- Awareness of the team's 'context and relationship to the organisation'.

(Adapted from Wake-Dyster, 2001, pp. 39–40)

Among the barriers to achieving success were short-term financial constraints that competed with longer-term quality improvements (Wake-Dyster, 2001). As we continue with this chapter you will realize that these are common themes underpinning the creation of successful interprofessional rehabilitation teams.

Research evidence can also help to highlight positive attributes of teams that have an impact on service-user care and recovery. Within the context of stroke rehabilitation for example, Strasser and colleagues (2005) evaluated the perceptions of 530 team members from 46 rehabilitation teams about team functioning on ten dimensions; they explored the association of these with functional improvement, discharge home and length of rehabilitation stay for service users. Three of the ten dimensions were associated with functional improvement, namely: (1) task orientation; (2) order and organization and (3) utility of quality information. One further dimension, team effectiveness, was associated with length of rehabilitation stay in quite a complex way: those teams that had high satisfaction with perceived effectiveness had patients with a longer mean length of stay, suggesting that these teams were better placed to advocate for longer hospitalizations and withstand pressures to discharge patients prematurely. In contrast, teams that had a strong sense of 'teamness' (which can be described as a sense of cohesion between team members) showed a trend towards reduced length of stay for their patients. It is not that one team was 'better' than the other, rather these results suggest the relationships between team effectiveness, efficiency and various patient outcomes are not straightforward and evaluations of teamwork need to take account of this complexity.

The tensions of working in teams

However, modern day teamwork is not without potential difficulties, for example Burton comments on the tensions between undertaking 'active therapy' and 'care components of nursing care' for nurses working in stroke units (Burton, 2000, p. 175). When professional boundaries are 'blurred' like this, it may be difficult for an individual professional to remain clear that they are operating within their scope of practice. The chapter co-author, Sarah, has developed a technique to overcome these tensions. For example she often starts a conversation by stating from which of her two professional stances she is operating, so as to make it clear from which background or skill set her contribution is coming from. Similarly there may be concerns regarding 'new types' of healthcare providers, such as the advanced or extended practice roles for allied health professionals mentioned earlier in this chapter. Murphy (2007) provides an interesting personal account of the medical profession's 'fears' that may be associated with such staff (namely that they will put existing doctors out of a job, will challenge the salaries and status of existing doctors, will result in other shortages in the workforce, or compete for private practice income if they move out of the publically funded service). It is likely that the changes in roles will continue apace because of impending workforce shortages, so Murphy concludes that it is important for doctors to overcome these fears and embrace change or even act as the champions or leaders of change (Murphy, 2007). What is interesting about the medical perspective of Murphy's article is that it reflects attitudes found by other researchers investigating collaborative practice: that doctors are less positive in their attitude towards teamwork and team training than nurses (Hansson et al., 2010). Further research is required to identify if the reasons for these attitudes lie in undergraduate training or elsewhere, such as in the tension between doctors' 'understanding of their professional role and their conditions of work' (Hansson et al., 2010, p. 84).

Sometimes the interprofessional working that we have been advocating in this book does not fit well with the requirements of professional registration simply because the very nature of interprofessional working is that it is about the overlapping of professional roles and responsibilities. For example, the UK's Health Professions Council requires professionals to meet standards regarding: character; health; proficiency (core competencies/benchmarked standards of practice); conduct, performance and ethics; and continuing professional development (CPD) (see www.hpc-uk.org/aboutregistration/standards/). There are also standards for education and training of the education providers, these standards relate to undergraduate training as well as CPD accredited courses and activities. However, conflict can arise when a CPD course offered by one professional body is not accepted as 'accredited' by a different professional body, which may create barriers to a professional wishing to acquire the skills usually attributed to another profession. The fitting together of standards and requirements for state registration, professional body membership and higher education course validation and accreditation is clearly complex. Some countries, such as the USA, have authorities for overseeing rehabilitation standards to help with this complexity (King et al., 2005).

Cleary these regulatory systems and standards are important for protecting the public. They also provide the basis for professional bodies or employing organizations to offer liability insurance or professional indemnity. This leads our debate on to the tensions and dilemmas that can arise from the legal implications of shared responsibility when practising in an interprofessional team.

Legal responsibilities arising from multidisciplinary meetings are brought into focus in the following example of a study that surveyed doctors' understanding of their individual accountability during team meetings about the care of patients with cancer (Sidhom and Poulsen, 2008). In the survey a description is given of a patient, aggrieved by a treatment decision made by a team and who wished to seek compensation; the question arising from this situation being who the court would consider responsible for the decision. The survey included questions about whether or not doctors were aware that they were individually accountable for the team decisions and whether the team meetings were conducted in such a way that reflected this individual responsibility. Based in four Australian tertiary care hospitals 18 teams and 136 doctors responded to the survey. It was clear that only 48% of doctors correctly thought they were individually liable; 33% felt that the team meeting environment was suboptimal for making decisions and on those occasions when doctors disagreed with a decision many did not formerly dissent at that time. The study authors concluded that doctors needed to be made aware of the legal implications of participating in multidisciplinary team meetings, with greater awareness of these responsibilities and improvements in the team dynamics being the way to 'optimize patient outcomes while limiting exposure of participants to legal liability' (Sidhom and Poulsen, 2008, p. 287). Unfortunately, this study did not involve other healthcare professionals but it does highlight the tensions that can occur within team decision-making situations.

In another study Nugus and colleagues describe how and where clinicians exercise power in their interprofessional relationships (Nugus et al., 2010). In this interactional study of health occupational relations the authors found two distinct types of power: collaborative or negotiated power versus competitive or authoritative power. It was not considered that one type was better but rather to what extent one type would be more appropriate than the other for a given context. The authors comment that the role of healthcare managers is to mediate between policy and practice but it may be that further research is needed to explore 'the interplay of managers in interprofessional relations, and to the challenges and opportunities of integrating care across formal service boundaries' (Nugus et al., 2010, p. 908).

Resolving these tensions at an individual level requires reflective practice that includes an awareness of personal and professional limitations and the development of skills for being a life-long learner. These are clearly necessary for keeping up-to-date in professional competencies. Resolving these tensions at a team level requires similar skills on the part of each team member but also processes and procedures within the team to help resolve conflict as well as a leader who knows when and how to move things on. Some of the basic principles for dealing with team conflict have been described by Anderson (2010) and the following is a synopsis of the main points:

- act in a timely way to identify the real points of difference, clarify the facts;
- get team members to resolve their differences, or compromise, based on these facts; or
- be prepared for the team leader to impose a resolution if needed.

Anderson (2010) also notes that not all disagreements are problematic, in fact healthy debate and constructive criticism should be encouraged. Allowing such debate but avoiding stand-offs is easier to achieve if the team is built and run effectively, as it is more likely that there will be trust and confidence in each other to cope with disagreements and any potentially damaging conflict can be dealt with promptly. A final point on this issue is that it may be appropriate to document the resolution and any action plans that arise from it.

Thinking outside the professional box

By now our understanding of what makes an effective interprofessional rehabilitation team as well as what tensions need to be overcome, is beginning to take shape. As a core theme for this book we acknowledge the contribution of many rehabilitation professionals, from differing backgrounds, who have informed our thinking, several of whom have been named at the start of this textbook. For example, a presentation given by Kath McPherson at the New Zealand Physiotherapy Conference (in Wellington, 2001) described a Venn diagram showing the intersection, or overlap, between discipline-specific knowledge and how transfer and accumulation of knowledge can lead to the production of deeper knowledge (see Figure 3.1). This deeper knowledge McPherson also describes as the 'new knowledge' of the team (McPherson et al., 2001; see also Gibbons et al., 1994).

Figure 3.1 is a way of illustrating how the whole can be greater than the sum of the parts. An effective rehabilitation team will then be able to use this new

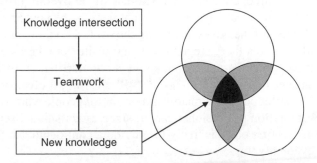

Figure 3.1 The active intersection of discipline-specific knowledge to produce new, 'deeper' knowledge of an interprofessional team. (Adapted and reproduced with permission from Kath McPherson.)

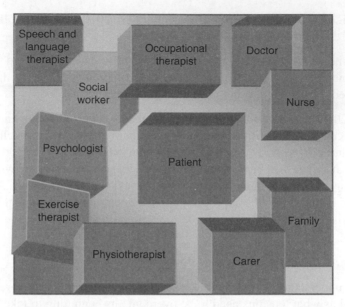

Figure 3.2   Thinking outside your professional box: an example of an interprofessional team where the whole is greater than the sum of the profession-specific parts.

knowledge in their practice, helping them to achieve what matters to the patient. Co-production of new knowledge is not only in relation to specific patients, but more broadly about rehabilitation theory and practice, thus it is perhaps one of the defining features of a successful interprofessional team. However, the concept requires individuals to move beyond their own professional boundaries and ways of thinking. True interprofessional working is a challenge, team members have to work to achieve this and have to develop the necessary teamwork skills. Taking these ideas into account we propose a 'thinking outside the professional box' model (see Figure 3.2) whereby each individual team member is represented by their own professional box but they all operate together within a bigger overall 'box'. This overall structure has a lot of 'new but shared space' that depicts the new knowledge of the team. We have shaded all the boxes, including the overall box, in various gradations of grey. This indicates that there are not black and white boundaries between members of the team but rather a gradient that could allow blurring, or even overlap of a boundary to a greater or lesser extent, while still allowing professional identity to remain intact. This latter point is probably important for people who are just embarking on their rehabilitation professional career, since establishing a sense of professional identity in the first place is likely to provide a confident base from which to work interprofessionally.

So our suggestion for 'thinking outside your professional box' is just that, to think beyond your own professional role and what might constitute not only other professionals' roles but also what is in the 'new shared space'. This 'thinking' is not the same as 'doing', as clearly each member of the team has to be confident that they are competent if they are to practice outside their professional box. Such additional competencies may require further training and development and possibly even insurance provision before they can be undertaken as part of the work you do for a team. For now all we ask is that you are prepared to keep an open mind about the grey area outside your professional 'box', as this thinking provides a strong basis for becoming interprofessional.

3.4 Team membership and roles

One approach to creating a team is to ensure all the relevant professions or disciplines are represented. As a starting point for informing who these relevant people might be we suggest that the International Classification of Functioning, Disability and Health (ICF, WHO, 2001) is used as a framework for identifying the right personnel. In Table 3.2 we show which people might be involved in rehabilitation of someone who has chronic low back pain by adapting a case mapping approach described by Allan et al. (2006).

This approach to defining who should be in the team makes intuitive sense providing all the required personnel are available, and there is one person who is always available but might not always be thought of as a team member: the patient or service user. This textbook contains a chapter dedicated to the service-user context (see Chapter 6) however, particular issues are thrown into sharp relief when reviewing the position of the service user within a rehabilitation team. Some of these issues relate to whether a service user is regarded as a team member, what 'power' or 'voice' the service user has, and to what degree this affects team dynamics.

In healthcare more generally the involvement of patients and the public in the development of services and the management of their own health conditions has been widely promoted (Department of Health, 2010; National Institute for Health and Clinical Excellence, 2011). Although initiatives for promoting the inclusion of patients and service users within rehabilitation service provision have been funded by the Department of Health, research shows that the rhetoric does not always match reality. Fudge et al. (2008) for example found that within the context of stroke rehabilitation, patient and public involvement tended to be initiated by professionals and that small numbers of service users were actually 'involved', so it seems unlikely that they would be considered members of the team. Fudge et al. conclude that the radical changes in services anticipated through greater engagement with the public and patients might be slow to occur. These authors call for greater debate about the rationale for service-user involvement, together with critical evaluation of the perceived benefits.

Other members of the team can be identified by their specialized role within the team as opposed to their professional contribution to the team. There are two specialized roles worth mentioning: the team leader role and the keyworker role. The latter role is described in Chapter 4, so here we will consider the skills that are required for team leadership.

Table 3.2 Identifying interprofessional team members using International Classification of Functioning, Disability and Health (ICF) terminology, the example of chronic low back pain.

Health condition:
Chronic low back pain

Body functions & structures:	Activity:	Participation:
Impairments of the spine and maybe lower limb e.g. movement range, strength, postural control, stamina and neurosensory systems. Rehabilitation approaches utilize: exercises to optimize muscular strength, power, co-ordination; medication; exercises and manual therapy techniques to increase range of movement and to reduce neurosensory symptoms. Team: patient, PT, pain specialist, psychologist	Limitations in tasks or actions e.g. sitting, getting up from sitting; bending, lifting, driving. Rehabilitation exercises will be task focused but tailored to individual activity limitations. Team: patient, PT, OT, exercise trainer, family	Restrictions to involvement in social, occupational or recreational life situations e.g. household duties, work, commuting to work, gardening, shopping, sport, community functions. Rehabilitation programme to address individual participation restrictions and create opportunities to participate in above roles. Team: patient, PT, OT, exercise trainer, social worker, occupational health physician/ nurse, friends and family
Environmental factors: Family, physical, social, occupational, attitudinal and other external contexts. Rehab addresses these factors by individually tailoring the programme and providing supplementary exercises or activity programme to perform at home. Team: patient, family and friends, employers/ occupational health staff, community PTs and OTs, GP		**Personal factors:** Age, gender, coping style, social background, education, profession, past and current experiences, behaviour patterns, character, attitudes and beliefs and other internal contexts. Rehab addresses some of these factors through cognitive–behavioural therapy or motivational counselling to decrease fear and anxiety and to improve confidence, performance mastery/self-efficacy and autonomy in ongoing rehabilitation. Team: patient, psychologist, OT, PT, friends and family

PT, physiotherapist; GP, general practitioner; OT, occupational therapist.

Team leadership

Leadership skills have been described extensively and numerous books on the topic can be found in any airport bookstore, from management and commerce literature to biographies about leaders throughout history (see for example Anderson, 2010). These can be useful for learning about the key principles of good leadership, however, we draw on resources from the rehabilitation literature to outline some of the essential characteristics of interprofessional team leadership (King et al., 2005; Wake-Dyster, 2001;) and our own experience of leading teams. The characteristics include personal attributes such as being able to:

- see the bigger picture, in particular an awareness of complexity at different levels (individual patient case level, team level, organizational level and funding/policy level);
- think creatively and inspire others to come up with innovative solutions;
- make timely or proactive decisions;
- communicate verbally and in written formats with clarity and precision;
- listen actively and be reflective;
- stay calm in pressurised situations;
- be objective and non-judgmental.

The team leader also needs a certain amount of knowledge, understanding and skills to manage a team effectively, these characteristics include:

- knowing the skills available from within the team;
- understanding team decision-making and problem-solving processes, including being able to negotiate compromises;
- ensuring team productivity and efficiency for example by keeping meeting discussions focused, clarifying roles and responsibilities, assigning timelines and deadlines;
- having knowledge of quality improvement and planning processes;
- being able to modify facilitation style and work with diversity, conflict and uncertainty;
- being able to motivate and influence, leading by example if appropriate;
- being willing to seek and provide support, ideas and learning opportunities for team members and team development;
- being willing to learn about leadership skills and how to facilitate team development.

(Adapted from King et al., 2005, Wake-Dyster, 2001)

There are numerous opportunities for developing leadership skills and many organizations provide courses for staff, from one-off in-house seminars through to extensive (and often expensive) programmes. We would encourage anyone aspiring to lead an interprofessional rehabilitation team to consider undertaking leadership training, particularly those courses that are designed to help you 'learn-in-action' – in other words a course that will support you while you are 'doing' leadership in your work. One of the authors, Claire, attended the Athena Programme for Executive Women, run by the Kings Fund charity (www.kingsfund.org.uk). This programme is delivered in four modules, over a 4- to 6-month period, supported by individual coaching in-between modules. The programme provides an opportunity for participants to reflect on challenges and issues emerging from 'real world' practice and implement new skills and strategies acquired during the programme with ongoing support and opportunities for review.

Specific team roles

In terms of professional contributions to a team there are occasions when some members of a team take on a specialized or extended role that is related to their scope of practice as well as to their role within the team. For example, teams may include physician assistants, nurse consultant practitioners or therapist consultants who may head up a specialist service like a stroke unit or an early supported discharge team. Similarly there are extended scope practitioners such as physiotherapists who work as orthopaedic clinic triage clinicians. With additional training these expert therapists can order X-rays and magnetic resonance imaging scans, their role enables a fast track assessment service for referral to either physiotherapy or further assessment for orthopaedic surgery (so cutting down waiting list times for orthopaedic consultation). Extended scope practitioners may also offer a specific treatment service (such as non-medics providing injections or medication prescriptions). These examples provide another dimension in considering what we mean by 'profession(al)' or 'discipline(ary)'. Beattie (1995) comments on the rule of purity versus the rule of relevance. 'Purity' in this sense means specialties that keep pure, true or honest to themselves and so create separate entities that keep things and people apart; sometimes pejoratively described as 'silos' of thinking and practice. In contrast 'relevance' refers to things that go together, a shared or common interest that results in collapsing and redrawing of boundaries; sometimes described as the 'generalist' approach. However, it should not be inferred that the 'generalist' lacks expertise, rather that they have been defined in a different way from that of the traditional 'pure' professional specialties. Thus, the consultant community therapist may have a generalist approach but at the same time be an expert in community-based rehabilitation practice. The following are some examples of the different ways in which rehabilitation personnel work in interprofessional teams:

- acute care teams;
- early supported discharge teams;
- complex care teams;
- community care teams;
- palliative care teams;
- integrated health and social care teams;
- intermediate care teams;
- hospital at home teams.

These are some of the different types of teams that have evolved over time in the UK; the particular constructions of the rehabilitation teams and how the team members practice often being shaped in response to wider political and societal agendas and funding environments.

In contrast another way of conceptualizing team roles and team members in rehabilitation is to consider the personal characteristics and preferences of individuals, rather than their profession, particularly in relation to shared activities, such as team meetings. For example, Belbin's team role theory has been influential within organizational psychology and management in facilitating this approach to teamwork (Belbin, 1981). An instrument known as Belbin's Team Role Self Perception Inventory (Furnham et al., 1993) can be used to help identify team roles, such as 'resource investigator' (keen to explore opportunities and develop contacts), 'co-ordinator' (who generally makes a good chairperson), 'teamworker' (who builds cohesion among members of the team) and 'completer-finisher' (who pays meticulous attention to detail, and perfects the final output).

There may, therefore, be various ways of determining the ideal skill set of a rehabilitation team. These may or may not be represented by conventional professional or disciplinary groups, roles or areas of practice. Clearly, there are rehabilitation professionals who regard their disciplinary or professional identity to be an important feature in describing their contribution and distinguishing their practice from that of others in the team. However, we have shown that there are alternative ways in which the constituent parts of an interprofessional team might be viewed and that there is not one 'ideal' team composition. Instead we suggest that a multilayered perspective of what makes up an interprofessional team allows the team to be responsive to service user needs and so enriches rehabilitation provision.

3.5 Processes of teamwork

Some of the specific processes that support teamwork in rehabilitation, such as goal planning, will be covered in detail in Chapter 4, so in this chapter we will focus on different activities associated with team practice in rehabilitation. These include shared assessment procedures, team meetings and team evaluation.

Interprofessional team assessment

An innovation in rehabilitation teamwork has been the advent of shared records and the use of the keyworker system (see also Chapter 4) to introduce the patient to the principles of rehabilitation and carry out an initial basic assessment of need. This mode of working is both cost effective for the team, in that essential information is elicited from the patient just once, and also avoids the patient having to take part in repeated interviews. In order for this system to be successful it is important that all members of the team share a commitment to this process. Van de Weyer et al. (2010), for example, found that in relation to goal setting in rehabilitation, some team members expressed the view that an initial meeting with the patient, in order to talk through the principles of goal setting, was viewed as being peripheral rather than a core element of treatment. The danger is then that efforts to understand the patient's perspective of their problems and their desired outcomes are subsumed within a desire to start 'hands on' treatment.

An important principle underpinning shared interprofessional assessment is the use of one theoretical framework to inform all aspects, including the initial meeting and any, more specialist, uni-professional aspects of assessment. As we have seen in Chapter 2 a model that has been used widely within rehabilitation assessment is the ICF (WHO, 2001). We suggest that the biopsychosocial perspective underpinning of the ICF does make it an excellent candidate for an overarching interprofessional assessment framework even if clinicians do not opt to use its full and very detailed assessment function. However, there are others, such as the Canadian Occupational Performance Model (Canadian Association of Occupational Therapists, 1997), which has already been briefly mentioned earlier in this chapter.

Another factor that is critical to good rehabilitation practice is the communication of the purpose, process and outcomes of assessment to the patient and, where appropriate, their family. This can sometimes be facilitated by enabling the patient to keep their own records, assessment reports etc and requires the use of appropriate language and formats to enable the patient to access the information recorded, including legible handwriting. Another method for facilitating communication is the use of team meetings.

Team meetings

The rehabilitation literature offers some guidance about how team meetings should be structured and run (see for example King et al., 2005, p. 1061) but there is little information about how frequently they should occur or who should attend. So instead it is perhaps more useful to work out a list of what might be the key requirements for successful team meetings to occur and then this list can be refined according to individual experiences and contexts. In Table 3.3 we provide such a list as a basis for this process.

The list in Table 3.3 is not exhaustive and clearly there does need to be some flexibility around the type of meetings that occur. One potentially different type of meeting is when there is a case conference or family meeting in which carers and/or members of the patient's immediate family attend the meeting. In Chapter 6 we cover some of the features of involving families in rehabilitation so the following will focus on the family meeting process. Family meetings can be especially useful when: (1) a specific purpose has been identified for the meeting (for example planning discharge home or reviewing long-term care arrangements); (2) those people who need to be there do actually attend, so the necessary people are present but there is not an overwhelming number of people attending; (3) the carer and family are given sufficient notice of the meeting and prepared for the purpose of the meeting (for example a written agenda could be provided in advance); (4) the meeting is well run (as for any team meeting, see Table 3.3); (5) meeting notes or minutes with any action plans are circulated to families, in a timely manner, after the meeting.

Table 3.3 Potential requirements for a successful team meeting.

Meeting preparation	Running the meeting	After the meeting
• Date and time arranged well ahead of meeting, to suit as many as possible • Date, venue and further details circulated well ahead of time • Room, phone conferencing etc arranged • Identified who is to attend (and how often) • Agenda or check list created • Roles identified (chair person, note taker etc) • Ground rules agreed (confidentiality, etiquette, use or no use of mobile phones, attendance and time keeping etc) • General structure of meeting established i.e. very structured versus flexible	• Starting on time, keeping to time, finishing on time • Clear leadership/chairperson • Clearly stated purpose/desired outcomes • Clearly stated interim goals or tasks • Outcomes/goals/tasks are achievable and specify realistic timeframes • Explicit and agreed assignment of actions: awareness of what is to be done and by whom • Reflection on whether the meeting focused on person who mattered (patient)	• Timely and appropriate methods for dissemination of team meeting information (prompt typing up and circulation of minutes) • Clear action points with dates and person responsible • Opportunity for querying or correcting minutes • Open communication about any challenges or issues in carrying out actions, which will facilitate learning • Progress monitoring and clarity about how this is assessed • Outcome evaluation and clarity about how this is assessed • Appropriate handling of failures (to meet outcomes) or conflict • Team housekeeping processes (team organization reviews, time for team development, conflict resolution training, dissemination processes established etc)

Clearly good communication with patients, their carers and families is crucial to successful rehabilitation practice and yet this is not always achieved. At this point it is worth considering if a formal family meeting is the best way to discuss rehabilitation plans with carers and other members of a family. For example, all parties coming to such a meeting may be apprehensive. From the staff perspective, they may not feel sufficiently skilled at dealing with confrontations (if they occur), they may resent the time away from their work with patients, especially if more time is required to explain 'taken for granted' medical terminology or to check that a person has a clear understanding of what is being discussed. Similarly, family members may also be anxious about the situation, not just because their loved one is unwell and there is some degree of uncertainty about their future, but also because they are overwhelmed by the number of people attending the meeting, their uniforms or professional status. In addition the setting may be an alien clinical environment, or just not conducive to a friendly discussion (e.g. cramped, hot room, people coming and going, bleeps going off, insufficient chairs and so on). There is also the likelihood that people come to the meeting with different preconceptions: relatives may worry that the meeting has been called because the patient is going to be discharged tomorrow, when this may not have been the intention at all. In addition, there may not be an appreciation by the family of the active, participative nature of rehabilitation, leading to misunderstandings about the role of the rehabilitation staff. There is a danger that the patient and their family can get too overawed to express their views or join in the discussion, leaving the health professionals in the situation of talking *at* them instead of *with* them. We also know that about only 40% of information is retained by patients from a single consultation (Ley, 1982) and this is likely to be true for family members attending meetings. This means much of the information has to be gone over again or given in additional ways before everyone is clear about what was covered in the meeting. In summary, it may just not be cost effective to run family meetings and instead other ways of involving the family are worth considering.

Alternatives include using the keyworker to discuss matters with the family (see also Chapter 4). It may be appropriate for the keyworker to talk to either a particular family member or several members. It may also be useful to arrange for one or two other team members to attend, so key people are present, but overall numbers are kept low. It may then be more likely that a smaller room can be arranged that provides an environment conducive to discussion and privacy. Another option could be to conduct the meeting by phone, at a pre-arranged time so that everyone 'books' the time into their schedule, this may be much more convenient for the family, especially if travel to and from the hospital is difficult or expensive. A further alternative for a team meeting can be achieved by accompanying the patient to a particular therapy session, when family members may also be present or have been specifically invited along. The decision to discharge someone with a disability back to their home or transferring them to a residential care home can be a difficult issue to raise and family members may need time to adjust to the idea. The informality of a one-to-one conversation may help the process of adjustment, people can raise their fears and concerns, as well as start to contemplate the changes that are about to take place. If needed, a bigger team meeting could then take place to discuss the practicalities of implementing any decision.

Team evaluation

A range of quality appraisal tools are available to help rehabilitation teams to enhance their processes through the evaluation of their team functioning. For example, the Rehabilitation Activities Profile (RAP) provides a method for improving patient-specific communication and record keeping among team members and aims to make team meetings much more efficient or streamlined. However, it is not clear what effect this has on actual rehabilitation outcomes (Beckerman et al., 2004). This is a common criticism of both team development activities and team evaluation tools. In Chapter 5 you will read more about measurement and evaluation in rehabilitation, so for now we will just make a couple of points related to this problem. The first is that it is likely to be very difficult to design an evaluation tool that is able to capture 'team effectiveness' as well as 'health outcomes' and second it may be more appropriate to regard 'team effectiveness' as a process by which 'health outcomes' can be achieved, hence the need for distinct evaluation tools and perhaps less expectation that one tool can do it all.

With this in mind we return to consider two more examples of team evaluation. The first example is the 'team survey', initially developed Millward and Ramsey in 1998 and then validated by Millward and Jeffries (2001). The tool comprises a number of different 'team dimensions: team potency, team identification, Shared Mental Models and team meta-cognition'. The authors were able to demonstrate reliability and validity of the tool from work involving ten teams (with 124 individuals) from a number of different locations in a large UK National Health Service (NHS) trust and representing teams from a wide range of specialities including management, service support and service delivery teams. They concluded that the tool is a 'robust and suitable tool for assessing health care team performance' (Millward and Jeffries, 2001, p. 284).

The second example is a project that is currently underway in the UK, called the 'EEICC Project: Enhancing the Effectiveness of Interprofessional Team Working'. The project is based at the University of Sheffield, School of Health and Related Research, it commenced in 2008 and is being led by Dr Susan Nancarrow. Set in community-based older peoples' services the project aims to optimize team working through the implementation of an Interprofessional Management Tool (IMT). The tool is under-pinned by three core themes that are considered to influence team performance:

• individual factors (motivation and satisfaction, career development, autonomy);
• team level factors (team size, integration, meetings, innovation);
• leadership factors (clarity, centralised/distributed, quality).

(Adapted from EEICC Project, 2011)

The project evaluation includes measures targeted at staff including leadership and workforce questionnaires, as well as separate measures to assess patient outcomes and to estimate the economic costs of implementing IMT. A presentation giving an interim progress report of the project indicates high satisfaction among the teams with the implementation process, which led to demonstrated improvements in team-work activities but an acknowledgement that it is still too early to assess patient and economic outcomes (Ariss, personal communication, 2011; see also www.sdo.nihr. ac.uk for the final project report). This again highlights the complexity of assessing teamwork, with considerable time being needed not only to do an evaluation of the team-building process but also for measuring subsequent health outcomes.

Regardless of how one decides to evaluate a team performance it is important to recognize that the team itself may be subject to a process of change or flux. Teams operate in a dynamic environment and so need to be able to develop and enhance their practice as well as evaluate their performance. This is particularly true given the rapid pace of change occurring both in healthcare generally and more specifically in the UK's NHS.

3.6   The role of interprofessional education in rehabilitation

Interprofessional education (IPED) has been developed and promoted for the past 50 years and a specific rehabilitation focus can be seen in the UK during the early 1990s when joint training programmes were established for physiotherapy and occupational therapy at the Universities of East Anglia and Southampton. Later, IPED in the UK

Table 3.4   Principles of interprofessional education: values. (Adapted from and including six statements reproduced from the Centre for the Advancement of Interprofessional Education (CAIPE) website by Barr and Low (2011) with permission from CAIPE.)

Values in interprofessional education	Achieved
• Focuses on the needs of individuals, families and communities to improve their quality of care, health outcomes and well-being • Applies equal opportunities within and between the professions and all with whom they learn and work • Respects individuality, difference and diversity within and between the professions and all with whom they learn and work • Sustains the identity and expertise of each profession • Promotes parity between professions in the learning environment • Instils interprofessional values and perspectives throughout uniprofessional and multiprofessional learning	• By keeping best practice central throughout all teaching and learning • By acknowledging but setting aside differences in power and status between professions • By utilizing distinctive contributions to learning and practice • By presenting each profession positively and distinctively • By agreeing 'ground rules' • By permeating means and ends for the professional learning in which it is embedded

moved on from just linking one or two related professions and extended to include virtually all the undergraduate health professional training programmes. One example is known as the New Generation project, a common learning approach in health and social care undergraduate education. This commenced in 2003 and involved over 2000 healthcare-related students based at the Universities of Southampton and Portsmouth and the local NHS (see O'Halloran et al., 2006). For those who are interested in exploring IPED further it is worth taking a look at the additional resources recommended at the end of this chapter, in particular the Centre for the Advancement of Interprofessional Education (CAIPE). This provides comprehensive information and offers the following definition of IPED that 'occurs when two or more professions learn with, from and about each other to improve collaboration and quality of care' (CAIPE, 2002, para. 1). Two key contributors, Hugh Barr and Helena Lowe have written about the principles for underpinning IPED. We have listed some of their values and how these can be achieved in Table 3.4. Many of these principles have direct relevance to practising rehabilitation teams as well as to those who are still in their undergraduate training.

We have already discussed some of the tensions related to interprofessional teamwork and there are some tensions arising from IPED as well. From experience of teaching on interprofessional programmes, the authors of this chapter can report that not all students see the relevance of learning about other professional groups. This can occur if a student is not clear about their own professional identity so finds it hard to convey what their role ought to be in an interprofessional team. In addition, students may feel their learning has to concentrate on learning about their own profession-specific skills and there is not enough time in the curriculum to do justice to this, let alone consolidate these skills. Furthermore, clinical training placements can mean that even if a student has embraced IPED they may find themselves in a situation where the senior clinical staff, who are supervising them, do not buy into the interprofessional model of practice. Although we are hopeful that such scenarios are diminishing in their prevalence there clearly remains some tension between traditional ways of practice for some staff and the 'new generation' of staff who aspire to interprofessional practice.

Despite these tensions, the literature is clear that IPED in general (i.e. broader than just for interprofessional rehabilitation) 'enables collaborative practice which in turn optimizes health-services, strengthens health systems and improves health outcomes' (WHO, 2010, p. 18). Most of this evidence arises from work that focuses on specific groups such as medical, dental and nursing professionals, or on specific patient populations such as those receiving mental health services, or treatment for heart failure (WHO, 2010). However, some evidence is also emerging for what might be considered as more rehabilitation-focused IPED. The following are three examples from around the world.

The first example, from Australia, is the team-link study based in primary care (Harris et al., 2010). The intervention was based on 'team care arrangements' and was designed to 'enhance communication and working relationships with service providers outside the general practice' (p. 8). The service providers were nurses and a wide range of allied health professionals (AHPs) working in the community and involved in the management of people with chronic illness (diabetes and cardiovascular disease). The results revealed that general practitioners (GPs) made changes to the way they managed patient care with some collecting more detailed patient histories in order to facilitate the development of patient care plans. The GPs also reported having a greater understanding of AHPs' roles and what information needed to be passed on to them, resulting in greater patient satisfaction with care. The GPs were also more confident in making referrals to AHPs. However, they also noted that it took a long time to build two-way trust and professional relationships and this 'required a strong commitment to teamwork' (Harris et al., 2010, p. 12). The authors concluded that it was feasible to facilitate team linking but that it was 'constrained by structural barriers to trust and communication' (such as geographical distance and funding arrangements) (p. 13).

The second example is a project based in Canada that utilized an assessment tool called SBAR (Situation Background Assessment Recommendation) to communicate falls risk and management in interprofessional teams (Velji et al., 2010). This was targeted for use by three groups of healthcare staff: those delivering direct patient care, unit leaders and support staff. A 'learning-in-action' approach was taken with SBAR being used as a communication tool to help improve the safety culture, team processes and team communication for an initiative called SAFE (Stop Adverse Falls Events). Key champions were identified to reinforce, encourage and model the use of SBAR and learning aids such as video and DVDs were used to help implementation. Evaluation of the project included a measure of team effectiveness called Team Survey (Millward and Jeffries, 2001) and safety reporting. The results indicated a reduction in 'near miss' falls and major falls. However, there was an overall increase in total number of falls, reflecting the fact that rehabilitation is inherently risky if we are to maximize people's functional ability. The authors identified there was a need to sustain the effects of the initiative; recognize the diversity of use for the SBAR tool (risk assessment, handovers, debriefing); make use of the implementation toolkit (video, DVD); and to consider using examples that were context and case relevant to reinforce learning (Velji et al., 2010).

The third example, from the UK, links interprofessional education and theory to clinical practice through the use of Action Research (which, in this example, involved in-depth and multiple perspectives being obtained in the clinical setting throughout the duration of the project). The study (Kilbride et al., 2010) involved 74 individuals who were all connected to the development of a stroke unit in a large London hospital where stroke care lacked co-ordination and was spread across a large number of wards. For example there were 22 nurses, 10 physiotherapists, 8 occupational therapists, 2 speech and language therapists, a ward clerk, a dietician and a volunteer service representative to name a few of the 20 staff groups taking part. The intention of the study was to create a Community of Practice, which is essentially the coming together of a group of people who share a common purpose or concern and who, by working together, also learn together about how to improve their practice (Wenger et al., 2002). A particularly important feature of a Community of Practice is that it is collegial and does not have a hierarchical structure (Bate and Robert, 2002). In the research study the stroke unit development process was supported by the implementation of a number of operational structures, such as team meetings, goal setting, joint treatment sessions, using whiteboards for team messages and so on. These structures reflect much of what we have been discussing in this chapter in terms of the characteristics that underpin interprofessional teamwork. The success of the development process was evaluated by tracking changes in the hospital's rating by the National Sentinel Stroke Audit; the scores moved from the bottom 5% (in 1998) to the top scoring service in 2004. However, the mechanisms by which this was achieved are also worth noting as again they reflect the processes by which good interprofessional practice can be achieved. For example: (1) top-down *and* bottom-up organizational engagement and involvement; (2) 'building and maintaining the team and its identity, valuing diversity and celebrating success'; (3) 'developing relationships, trust and social capital'; (4) 'recognising and valuing' that the nurse has a central role in stroke care; (5) 'protected time for team members to reflect, plan and work together'; (6) 'making learning an everyday occurrence'; and (7) 'the utility of vertical and horizontal organizational links' (Kilbride et al., 2010, p. 7).

These three examples all demonstrate how IPED and research can help facilitate interprofessional teamwork in the rehabilitation practice setting.

3.7   Collaborative rehabilitation research

Interdisciplinary working is also an important feature of applied health research and there has been a strong push for involving patients, carers and the public in such research. The meaningful inclusion of service users in designing and evaluating rehabilitation services more widely is also gathering increasing support.

In order to support this development INVOLVE, a national UK organization, has been established by the Department of Health to promote patient and public involvement (PPI) in health and social care research, including the design, commissioning, evaluation and dissemination of research (see www.involve.org.uk). For example a research study was recently funded through the National Institute of Health Research (NIHR) programme called 'Research for Patient Benefit' on which one of the chapter authors, Claire was a co-applicant along with Susan, a lay representative. Susan became a co-applicant on this project by virtue of her role as a carer, and contributed to the design of the project (focusing on evaluation of services for people with dementia) including suggestions for the intervention. Susan's time prior to submission of the research funding application was recompensed by the NIHR Research Design Service South Central, using guidelines produced by INVOLVE (INVOLVE, 2009). Susan remains involved with the project, with her contribution included as part of the overall costs that will be supported by the research award.

An example of successful interdisciplinary research collaboration with the potential to impact on interprofessional rehabilitation practice is the Going Outdoors: Falls, Ageing and Resilience (or Go Far) programme. This research is funded through a strategic grant from the Medical Research Council's Lifelong Health and Wellbeing initiative (itself a cross-council initiative to support multidisciplinary research exploring healthy ageing and wellbeing – see http://www.mrc.ac.uk/Ourresearch/ResearchInitiatives/ LLHW/index.htm). The collaboration is led by a professor with expertise in the design of the built and urban environment for older people and the research co-applicants include an occupational therapist (Claire), psychologists, gerontologists and an exercise physiologist. Through a series of work packages the programme aims to:

- explore the role of the outdoor environment in shaping inequalities in health;
- explore older people's views and experiences of falling outdoors;
- develop strategies to evaluate the relationship between the older person and the outdoor environment;
- develop a plan for future cross-disciplinary research in this area.

A number of interesting issues have arisen from this collaboration. First, a shared understanding about what constitutes rigorous research methodologies and methods for all disciplines needed to be developed. Second, meaningful and valued outputs had to be agreed. Third, preferred methods of communication had to be established. Fourth, the degree of (in)formality and importance attached to user involvement had to be acknowledged and accepted. One of the aspirations of the programme is to reflect upon the process of collaboration in order to see what can be learnt about successful joint working.

3.8   The future for interprofessional rehabilitation teams

One fairly clear way of taking interprofessional rehabilitation forward is to use the framework of the ICF to inform our thinking. If all professional groups are versed in the domains of the ICF and understand the conceptual underpinning, namely the biopsychosocial model and the move away from impairment-driven healthcare, then there is likely to be some common ground for sharing our approach to rehabilitation practices. Similarly the ICF provides a language and terminology that can be shared, allowing communication between different professional groups to occur in a smooth and clear manner. If we are all aware of the goal of overcoming participation restrictions or that there can be a tendency to revert to a focus on impairments then checks and balances can be made to realign practice or a professional's approach to what really matters for the patient. Allan and colleagues (2006) propose 'a conceptual model for interprofessional education' that utilizes the ICF framework to help students to operationalize the underpinning biopyschosocial model. These authors use the example of an elderly gentleman with complex health problems including stroke and diabetes, to illustrate how the case details can be listed in accordance with the ICF domains with arrows linking each list to the corresponding part of the ICF diagram. This is similar in principle to the way we mapped the low back pain case in Table 3.2, although we have taken Allan et al.'s mapping approach a step further by embedding the case details into the actual ICF diagram. Allan and colleagues (2006) suggest this mapping activity is particularly useful for complex cases, introducing students to a 'holistic and inclusive' approach and opportunities to learn about other disciplines. They conclude that 'the language of the ICF provides a common ground for interprofessional and international communication' and 'a strong foundation in the principles exemplified by the ICF may serve to enhance interprofessional communication and learning, and in so doing, encourage involvement in interprofessional care' (Allan et al., 2006).

3.9 Conclusion

In this chapter we have discussed a number of different issues relating to interprofessional rehabilitation, from some of the terminology used to describe the team through to some of the characteristics of good teamwork and whether interprofessional teams are effective in delivering rehabilitation. We suggest that interprofessional rehabilitation can be achieved and that by using the framework of the ICF to inform our practice and by sharing the language of the ICF to facilitate our communication, we can start to think outside our professional box and operate in an interprofessional manner. This does not mean practising outside our competencies but it does, we propose, result in the interprofessional whole being greater than the sum of the profession-specific parts.

Additional resources

Centre for the Advancement of Interprofessional Education (CAIPE): www.caipe.org.uk (accessed 15 February 2012).

The Canadian Interprofessional Health Collaborative: http://www.cihc.ca/ (accessed 15 February 2012).

Australian Interprofessional Practice and Education Network (AIPPEN): http://www.aippen. net/ (accessed 15 February 2012).

European Interprofessional Education Network in Health and Social Care: http://www.eipen. org (accessed 15 February 2012).

The *Journal of Interprofessional Care* Common Learning: https://www.commonlearning.net/ project/index.asp (accessed 15 February 2012).

Finlay, L. and Ballinger, C. (2007). The challenge of working in teams. In: S. Fraser and S. Matthews (Editors). *The Critical Practitioner in Social Work and Health Care*. Los Angeles, CA: Sage Publications.

References

Allan, C. M., Campbell, W. N., Guptill, C. A., Stephenson, F. F. and Campbell, K. E. (2006). A conceptual model for interprofessional education: the International Classification of Functioning, Disability and Health (ICF). *Journal of Interprofessional Care*, *20*(3), 235–245.

Anderson, M. (2010). *The Leadership Book*. Harlow: Pearson Education.

Ariss, S. (2011). *Enhancing the Effectiveness of Interprofessional Team Working Project Presentation*, September 2011, Sheffield. Southampton: NIHR. http://www.sdo.nihr.ac.uk/ projdetails.php?ref=08-1819-214 (accessed 20 November 2011).

Ballinger, C. and Payne, S. (2002). The construction of the risk of falling among and by older people. *Ageing and Society*, *22*(3), 305–324.

Baptiste, M. L. S., Carswell, A., McColl, M. A., Polatajko, H. and Pollock, N. (2005). *Canadian Occupational Performance Measure (COPM)*, *(4th edn)*. Ottawa: CAOT Publications.

Barnard, S. and Wiles, R. (2001). Evidence-based physiotherapy. *Physiotherapy*, *87*, 115–124.

Barr, H. and Low, H. (2011). *Principles of Interprofessional Education*. Fareham: Centre for the Advancement of Interprofessional Education (CAIPE). www.caipe.org.uk (accessed 19 October 2011).

Bate, S. P. and Robert, G. (2002). Knowledge management and communities of practice in the private sector: lessons for modernizing the National Health Service in England and Wales. *Public Administration*, *80*(4), 643–663.

Beattie, A. (1995). War and peace among health tribes. In: K. Soothill, L. Mackay and C. Webb. (Editors). *Interprofessional Relations in Health Care*. London: Edward Arnold.

Beckerman, H., Roelofsen, E., Knol, D. L. and Lankhorst, G. J. (2004). The value of the Rehabilitation Activities Profile (RAP) as a quality sub-system in rehabilitation medicine. *Disability and Rehabilitation*, *26*(7), 387–400.

Belbin, M. (1981). *Management Teams*. London: Heinemann.

Boon, H., Verhoef, M., O'Hara, D. and Findlay, B. (2004). From parallel practice to integrative health care: a conceptual framework. *BMC Health Services Research*, *4*(15), 1–5. www.biomedcentral.com/1472-6963/4/15 (accessed 29 February 2012).

Browner, C. M. and Bessire, G. D. (2004). Developing and implementing transdisciplinary rehabilitation competencies. *Spinal Cord Injury Nursing*, *21*(4), 198–205.

Burton, C. R. (2000). A description of the nursing role in stroke rehabilitation. *Journal of Advanced Nursing*, *32*(1), 174–181.

Canadian Association of Occupational Therapists. (1997). *Enabling Occupation: An Occupational Therapy Perspective*. Ottawa: CAOT Publications.

Centre for the Advancement of Interprofessional Education (CAIPE). (2002). *Defining IPE*. Fareham: CAIPE. http://www.caipe.org.uk/about-us/defining-ipe (accessed 14 February 2012).

Dharm-Datta, S., Etherington, J., Mistlin, A., Rees, J. and Clasper, J. (2011). The outcome of British combat amputees in relation to military service. *Injury, 42*(11), 1362–1367.

Department of Health. (2010). *Equity and Excellence: Liberating the NHS*. Norwich: The Stationery Office.

Dillingham, T. R. (2002). Physiatry, physical medicine, and rehabilitation: historical development and military roles. *Physical Medicine and Rehabilitation Clinics of North America, 13*(1), 1–16.

Drinka, T. and Clark, P. (2000). *Health Care Teamwork: Interdisciplinary Practice and Teaching*. Westport, CT: Auburn House.

EEICC Project (2011). *The EEICC Project: Enhancing the Effectiveness of Interprofessional Team Working*. Sheffield: University of Sheffield www.sheffield.ac.uk/scharr/sections/hsr/rrg/eeicc/imt (accessed 20 November 2011).

Esnouf, J. E., Taylor, P. N., Mann, G. E. and Barrett, C. L. (2010). Impact on activities of daily living using a functional electrical stimulation device to improve dropped foot in people with multiple sclerosis, measured by the Canadian Occupational Performance Measure. *Multiple Sclerosis, 16*(9), 1141–1147.

Fudge, N., Wolfe, C. D. A. and McKevitt, C. (2008). Assessing the promise of user involvement in health service development: ethnographic study. *British Medical Journal 336*, 331.

Furnham, A., Steele, H. and Pendleton, D. (1993). A psychometric assessment of the Belbin Team-Role Self-Perception Inventory. *Journal of Occupational and Organizational Psychology, 66*(3), 245–257.

Gibbons, M., Limoges, C., Nowotny H., Schwartzman, S., Scott, P. and Trow, M. (1994). *The New Production of Knowledge: The Dynamics of Science and Research in Contemporary Societies*. London: Sage.

Guzzo, R. A. and Shea, G. P. (1992). Group performance and intergroup relations in organizations. In: *Handbook of Industrial and Organizational Psychology (2nd edn, Vol. 3)*. Palo Alto, CA: Consulting Psychologists Press, pp. 269–313.

Hansson, A., Arvemo, T., Marklund, B., Gedda, B. and Mattson, B. (2010). Working together – primary care doctors' and nurses' attitudes to collaboration. *Scandinavian Journal of Public Health, 38*, 78–85.

Harris, M. F., Chan, B. C., Daniel, C., Wan, Q., Zwar, N. and Powell-Davies, G. (2010). Development and early experience from an intervention to facilitate teamwork between general practices and allied health providers: the Team-link study. *BMC Health Services Research, 10*, 104.

Herbert, R. D., Maher, C. G., Moseley, A. M. and Sherrington, C. (2001). Effective physiotherapy. *British Medical Journal, 323*, 788–790.

Holliday, R. C., Ballinger, C. and Playford, E. D. (2007). Goal setting in neurological rehabilitation: Patients' perspectives. *Disability and Rehabilitation, 29*(5), 389–394.

INVOLVE. (2009). *Exploring Impact: Public Involvement in NHS, Public Health and Social Care Research*. London: INVOLVE.

Kilbride, C., Perry, L., Flatley, M., Turner, E. and Meyer, J. (2010). Developing theory and practice: creation of a community of practice through action research produced excellence in stroke care. *Journal of Interprofessional Care, 25*(2), 91–97.

King, J. C., Nelson, R. T., Blankenship, K. J., Turturro, T. C. and Beck, A. J. (2005). Rehabilitation team function and prescriptions, referrals and order writing. In: J. A. DeLisa (Editor-in-chief). *Physical Medicine and Rehabilitation Principles and Practice* (4th edn, Vol. 2). Philadelphia, PA: Lippincott Williams and Wilkins, pp. 1051–1072.

Ley, P. (1982). Satisfaction, compliance and communication. *British Journal of Clinical Psychology, 21*, 241–254.

Medical Research Programme. (2011) *Lifelong Health and Wellbeing*. London: MRC http://www.mrc.ac.uk/Ourresearch/ResearchInitiatives/LLHW/index.htm (accessed 22 November 2011).

McPherson, K. M., Headrick, L. A. and Moss, F. (2001). Working and learning together: good quality care depends on it, but how can we achieve it? *Quality and Safety in Healthcare, 10*(suppl. II), 46–53.

Millward, L. J. and Jeffries, N. (2001). The team survey: a tool for health care team development. *Journal of Advanced Nursing, 35*(2), 276–287.

Murphy, B. (2007). Medical role substitutions and delegations – overcoming the fear. *Australian Health Review, 31*(supplement 1), S20–S24.

National Institute for Health and Clinical Excellence. (2011). *Patient and Public Involvement Policy*. London: Nice. http://www.nice.org.uk/getinvolved/patientandpublicinvolvement/patientandpublicinvolvementpolicy/patient_and_public_involvement_policy.jsp?domedia=1andmid=5D00F560-19B9-E0B5-D48225F724082ED8 (accessed 22 November 2011).

Nugus, P., Greenfield, D., Travaglia, J., Westbrook, J. and Braithwaite, J. (2010). How and where clinicians exercise power: interprofessional relations in health care. *Social Science and Medicine, 71*, 898–909.

O'Halloran, C., Hean, S., Humphris, D. and Macleod-Clark, J. (2006). Developing common learning: the new generation project undergraduate curriculum model. *Journal of Interprofessional Care, 20*(1), 12–28.

Potter, J. (1996). *Representing Reality Discourse, Rhetoric and Social Construction*. London: Sage Publications.

Sidhom, M. A. and Poulsen, M. G. (2008). Group decisions in oncology: doctors' perceptions of the legal responsibilities arising from multidisciplinary meetings. *Journal of Medical Imaging and Radiation Oncology, 52*, 287–292.

Strasser, D. C. Falconer, J. A., Herrin, J. S., Bowen, S. E., Stevens, A. B. and Uomoto, J. (2005). Team functioning and patient outcome in stroke rehabilitation. *Archives Physical Medicine Rehabilitation, 86*, 403–409.

Townsend, E. A. and Polatajko, H. J. (2007). *Enabling Occupation II: Advancing an Occupational Therapy Vision for Health, Well-being and Justice through Occupation*. Ottawa: CAOT Publication.

Van de Weyer, R. C., Ballinger, C. and Playford, E. D. (2010). Goal setting in neurological rehabilitation: Staff perspectives. *Disability and Rehabilitation, 32*(17), 1419–27.

Velji, K., Baker, G.R., Fancott, C., Tardif, G., Aimone, E., Solway, S., Andreoli, A., Szeto, P., Hernandez, C. and Holdsworth, S. (2010). *Using SBAR to Communicate Falls Risk and Management in Interprofessional Rehabilitation Teams*. Edmonton: Canadian Patient Safety Institute.http://www.patientsafetyinstitute.ca/English/research/cpsiResearchCompetitions/2007/Documents/Velji/Report/Velji%20and%20Baker%20Full%20Report.pdf (accessed 20 November 2011).

Wade, D. T. (2000). Personal context as a focus for rehabilitation. *Clinical Rehabilitation, 14*, 115–118.

Wade, D. T. and de Jong, B.A. (2000). Recent advances in rehabilitation. *British Medical Journal, 320*, 1385–1388.

Wake-Dyster, W. (2001). Designing teams that work. *Australian Health Review*, 24(4), 34–41.

Walker, L. O. and Avant, K. C. (1995). *Strategies for Theory Construction in Nursing (3rd edn)*. Norwalk, CT: Appleton and Lange.

Wenger, E., McDermott, R. and Snyder, W. M. (2002). *A Guide to Managing Knowledge Cultivating Communities of Practice*. Boston, MA: Harvard Business School Publishing.

World Health Organization. (2001). *International Classification of Functioning, Disability and Health: ICF*. Geneva: World Health Organization.

World Health Organization. (2010). *The Framework for Action on Interprofessional Education & Collaborative Practice*. Geneva: WHO.

Yardley, L., Beyer, N., Hauer, K., McKee, K., Ballinger, C. and Todd, C. (2007). Recommendations for promoting the engagement of older people in activities to prevent falls. *Quality and Safety in Health Care*, 16(3), 230–234.

Chapter 4

Processes in rehabilitation

William Levack[1] and Sarah G. Dean[2]

[1]*Associate Dean, Research and Postgraduate Studies for the University of Otago Wellington and Senior Lecturer in Rehabilitation for the Rehabilitation Teaching and Research Unit, Department of Medicine, University of Otago Wellington, New Zealand;* [2]*Senior Lecturer in Health Services Research, University of Exeter Medical School, United Kingdom*

4.1   Introduction

Clinical rehabilitation is frequently described as being a 'process' (Wade, 2005). The word 'process' is used in this context to emphasize the idea that rehabilitation is largely a problem-solving activity rather than collections of techniques implemented in response to pre-specified presenting conditions. Rehabilitation seldom involves following a fixed decision-making algorithm. Instead, rehabilitation professionals aim to work on an individual basis with the patients in their services to identify and address key factors that restrict their ability to engage fully in the activities and social roles of their daily life.

Providers of rehabilitation services learn a wide range of different types of interventions for common conditions. These interventions may be highly technical or specific to their professional disciplines: exercise prescription for movement retraining or cardiovascular fitness; manufacturing individually crafted splints for positioning parts of the body; cognitive–behaviour therapy; tendon transfer surgery; teaching self-catheterization; adapting environments for work or home life; providing assistive technology; teaching strategies for energy conservation; prescribing medication for various physical or psychological impairments and so on. Indeed, medical libraries are full of textbooks providing detailed information about many such interventions, techniques and strategies for specific professional groups, specific patient populations or specific areas of clinical practice. However, regardless of the exact context of any one rehabilitation service, four major components are always central to rehabilitation process:

- assessment (diagnosis and the collection of data for rehabilitation planning);
- goal planning (identification and prioritization of the objectives of rehabilitation);

Interprofessional Rehabilitation: A Person-Centred Approach, First Edition.
Edited by Sarah G. Dean, Richard J. Siegert and William J. Taylor.
© 2012 John Wiley & Sons, Ltd. Published 2012 by John Wiley & Sons, Ltd.

- interventions (specific actions or activities);
- evaluation (comparing actual and planned outcomes).

(Wade et al., 2010)

Together these components form a process that has been called the 'rehabilitation cycle' (Wade, 2005; Rauch et al., 2008). A typical representation of this cycle is of a circle (Wade, 2005): one that starts from entry into the rehabilitation service with an assessment, leading through to goal setting and interventions, to evaluation of outcomes, and onwards to discharge from the service or re-assessment if problems have not resolved (see Figure 4.1). However a more accurate representation of the rehabilitation cycle for many situations, particularly those involving long-term or complex disability, is probably that of a spiral (see Figure 4.2). This is because each round of the 'cycle' can lead to changes in a number of variables that alter what might be considered the best direction or best end-point for an individual's episode of rehabilitation. Such variables include an individual's prognosis for improvement (which can be viewed as better or worse than initially expected as a result of actual progress), the values or goals of the patients and their family (which can change as a result of learning more about the nature of their condition or if their experience of disability and recovery alters what they consider most important), or the emergence of new opportunities (that arise as a result of changes in a person's functional capacity or social and environmental support).

This chapter provides an overview of each of the four key components of the rehabilitation process with an emphasis on how these are linked through goal planning. Also introduced in this chapter are other concepts related to the process of rehabilitation: keyworking, motivation, adherence, engagement of the patient in the rehabilitation process and transitions from hospital to the community.

4.2   Assessment

The rehabilitation process begins with assessment of the person admitted to the service. Typically, as rehabilitation is often a post-acute service, patients arrive at rehabilitation with a written or oral referral from another health professional or health funder. These referrals are likely to contain information about the person's presenting condition and relevant clinical history. However, it is highly important that further information is gathered before planning a course for rehabilitation.

Assessment in a rehabilitation context needs to be *holistic*. This often over-used word simply means that when gathering information about a patient for the purposes of planning rehabilitation, the assessment process needs to provide a complete overview of that person. This includes not only collection of information about all aspects of their physical, psychological and social health, but also collection of information on the following:

- The environmental and social context of their usual life outside of the rehabilitation service;

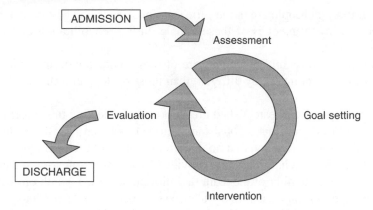

Figure 4.1 The rehabilitation cycle.

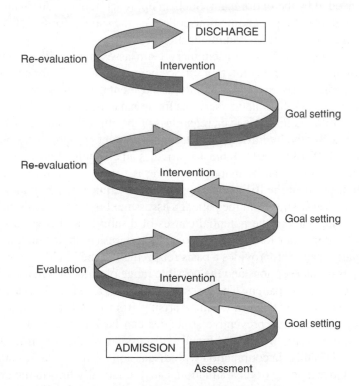

Figure 4.2 Alternative rehabilitation cycle – the rehabilitation spiral.

- their expectations of the rehabilitation service and objectives for the future;
- who they are as individuals (i.e. what they value, their interests, their sociocultural background and their personal strengths);
- what their understanding is of their health and disability (i.e. what they perceive to be the cause of any current difficulties they might have in their life, what they believe needs to occur to address these difficulties, what their expectations are for recovery);

- who the important people are in their life (family, friends and advocates), and what the expected involvement is of these people during rehabilitation and following discharge;
- what the expectations and objectives are of these other important people (which may be similar to or markedly different than those of the patient).

Assessment templates and established procedures for collecting this information can be very helpful to ensure that a consistent approach is taken for all people entering into a rehabilitation service and that no important aspects of the assessment are omitted by mistake. When rehabilitation is provided by an interprofessional team, it can be beneficial if one member of the team (a senior nurse, allied health professional or doctor) conducts an interdisciplinary team assessment (see also Chapter 3). This assessment would include collection of all the basic health and contextual information that is needed by the entire team. Such an approach reduces duplication (avoiding several team members spending time collecting the same information on multiple occasions) and improves team communication.

The exact content of an interdisciplinary team assessment will of course differ depending on the type of rehabilitation service being provided. Different types of services (e.g. paediatric services, community-based mental health services, outpatient pain clinics, inpatient rehabilitation services for spinal cord injury etc.) all require different types of information. However, regardless of the clinical context, it can be useful to structure much of the interdisciplinary team assessment around the framework provided by the ICF (WHO, 2001). Table 4.1 provides an example of how components of the assessment process can be mapped onto the ICF framework (see Chapter 2 for more information about the ICF and its application to clinical rehabilitation).

The information arising from the patient's assessment is used in a number of ways. It informs the team about the potential causes of disability and areas where further gains are needed in order for the patient to make progress in their functional abilities and social participation. It provides a basis for predicting the likelihood of success of different types of interventions and the possible range of outcomes that could reasonably be expected for the patient. The assessment process also identifies areas where a patient is at risk of further harm (such as arising from pressure areas, urinary tract infections or falls) so that preventive strategies can be implemented to reduce the chances of these events occurring. Finally, discussion of the assessment with the patient and their family, in conjunction with discussion of their values, hopes, expectations, and understanding of their situation, can dramatically inform the goal-setting process, which is central to good rehabilitation planning.

Organizing the interdisciplinary team to undertake their assessment can sometimes be usefully incorporated into the role of a *keyworker* (or *case manager*), whereby one member of the team becomes the central point for contact and communication between the patient, their family and the interprofessional rehabilitation team (see also Chapter 3). In addition to the interdisciplinary team assessment, the keyworker can also meet regularly with the patient and their family to explain the rehabilitation process, set and revise goals, discuss the patient's progress and present the team's

Table 4.1 Matching assessment components to the International Classification of Functioning, Disability and Health (ICF) (WHO, 2001).

ICF component	Examples of assessment components
Health condition Body structures and functions	Diagnosis (or diagnoses) Arousal Physiological function (e.g. blood pressure, heart rate, respiratory rate, blood tests, urinalysis) Pain Muscle strength Range of movement Neurological symptoms (e.g. reflexes, spasticity) Sensory function (e.g. sensation, vision, hearing) Nutritional status Eating or swallowing difficulties Skin integrity and wounds Cognition (e.g. memory, orientation, awareness, concentration, perception) Communication Continence Sexual function
Activity limitations	Mobility Self-cares (bathing, grooming, toileting, dressing/undressing) Risk of falls Managing finances Driving
Participation	Social roles in the home Social roles in the community Work or training status
Environmental factors	Residential situation Work environment Disability support services being received Medications Assistive technology used Respiratory support used Family/friend involvement Family/friend attitudes and beliefs Legal status (e.g. power of attorney)
Personal factors	Age Gender Ethnicity Religion Vocational identity Self-identity Personal attitudes and beliefs

perspectives on the likely outcomes from further clinical intervention. The keyworker can also invest time to find out more about the patient and family's expectations for interventions and recovery, about any concerns they might have about the patient's health and well-being or services received, and can report this information back to the rest of the rehabilitation team. Furthermore, the keyworker can take responsibility for the overall coordination of the rehabilitation process for that individual, directing the rehabilitation planning for the team and ensuring that it is carried out in a timely fashion. In some teams, the keyworker is the one who chairs the team meetings or family meetings when that particular patient is discussed (see Chapter 3 for more about team meetings).

4.3   Goal planning

Early in the rehabilitation process, goals should be set to direct the course of rehabilitation interventions (or at the very least, to make explicit the intended outcome of the rehabilitation service for the individual patient). Some have presented goal planning as a relatively simple, straightforward way of interacting with patients in order to prioritize interventions, facilitate teamwork and improve health outcomes (Wilson, 2008). However, increasingly it has become apparent that multiple approaches to goal planning exist (see Table 4.2), involving a variety of procedures and serving a

Table 4.2   A list of approaches to goal setting.

Approach to goal setting	References
Goal attainment scaling	Original version: Kiresuk and Sherman (1968) Contemporary approaches: Turner-Stokes (2009); Turner-Stokes and Williams (2010)
Goal setting based on the Canadian Occupational Performance Measure	Pendleton and Schultz-Krohn (2005); Phipps and Richardson (2007); Trombly et al. (2002); Wressle et al. (2002)
'SMART' goal planning	Barnes and Ward (2000); Mastos et al. (2007); McLellan (1997); Monaghan et al. (2005); Schut and Stam (1994); Bovend'Eerdt et al. (2009)
'RUMBA' goal planning	Barnett (1999)
Self-identified goal assessment	Melville et al. (2002)
Goal management training	Levine et al. (2000)
The Rivermead Life Goals Questionnaire and approaches to goal planning from Rivermead Rehabilitation Centre	McGrath and Davis (1992); McGrath et al. (1995); Wade (1999a & b)
Approaches to goal planning from the Wolfson Neurorehabilitation Centre	McMillan and Sparkes (1999)
Contractually organized goal setting	Powell et al. (2002)
Collaborative goal technology	Clarke et al. (2006)
Goal setting as part of the Progressive Goal Attainment Programme	Sullivan et al. (2006)
Patient-centred functional goal planning	Randall and McEwen (2000)
Goal setting based on the Patient Goal Priority Questionnaire or Patient Goal Priority List	Åsenlöf and Silijebäck (2009)

RUMBA, Relevant, Understandable, Measurable, Behavioural and Achievable; SMART, Specific, Measurable, Achievable, Relevant, and Time-limited (but see text for alternative definitions).

range of different, sometimes conflicting functions (Levack et al., 2006a, 2006b; Playford et al., 2000). In this section an overview of common approaches to goal planning for rehabilitation has been provided. This overview is intended as a guideline only. Rehabilitation teams and individual health professionals are advised to tailor their approach to goal planning for the specific needs of their patients and the objectives of their services, drawing on relevant goal theory and research wherever possible.

What is a rehabilitation goal?

All human behaviour is arguably goal directed and, in its broadest sense, the term 'goal' can include a wide range of concepts – from biological goals (e.g. to change one's body temperature or reproduce) to complex, cognitive or aesthetic goals (such as to live a moral life or achieve a career objective); from goals that relate to a moment in time and goals that relate to a lifespan (Austin and Vancouver, 1996). In the context of rehabilitation however, the term 'goal' is generally used to mean something much more specific; more explicitly linked to clinical work. Rehabilitation goals are *usually* characterized by the following:

- reference to a desired future state that the patient cannot currently achieve;
- having the patient as the subject of the goal (e.g. 'that John will have no episodes of incontinence of urine over a 48-hour period within 2 weeks' as opposed to 'That the nurses will take John to the toilet every 4 hours' – the latter being an example of an 'action plan' or 'intervention');
- an emphasis on achievement at the level of activity and participation rather than body function and structure (e.g. 'that John will transfer independently from his bed to his wheelchair within 2 weeks' as opposed to 'that John will lift his leg against gravity with the knee straight while in supine lying within 2 weeks');
- an emphasis on outcomes to be achieved as a result of clinical interventions or the patient's effort, rather than as a result of the passage of time or natural healing and recovery;
- being explicit rather than implicit (i.e. explicit goals being those goals that the clinical staff and, usually, the patient and other involved people, such as their family, are consciously aware of; as opposed to implicit goals that have not been consciously expressed).

Regarding this last point, the act of reaching for a cup is a motor activity with an implicit goal (i.e. to take the cup). Asking a patient to reach for a cup (versus just asking them to reach into mid-air) is an example of using implicit goals to influence behaviour (Trombly and Wu, 1999) as the goal of taking a cup changes the kinematics of a reaching motion. However, using such activities as a clinical intervention (e.g. for exercise therapy after a stroke) is not an example of 'goal setting' in rehabilitation in its usual sense. Therefore while these types of 'task goals' are goals in the psychological sense, they are not examples of 'rehabilitation goals' as such. To make 'independently using a cup to drink' the subject of a 'rehabilitation goal', clinicians would have to explicitly set this as a goal, using some form of clinical documentation and only after discussion and negotiation of this as a goal of therapy with the patient.

Of course, exceptions to all of these general rules do exist. For instance, patients who have impairments related to orientation, memory or communication may not be explicitly aware of goals that their clinicians and family are working on or may only have limited capacity to participate in goal selection. Goals related to body function and structure (e.g. range of movement, muscle strength, respiratory status) may sometimes be useful to set in certain contexts – particularly in the early days of recovery from a very severe injury or illness, when goals related to activity or social participation may not be as meaningful. Some clinicians and their patients may also feel that it is valuable from the context of family-centred practice to set goals featuring family members as the subject of the goal (Levack et al., 2009), although others have argued that only patients should be the subject of goals, and never the significant other people in their lives (McMillan and Sparkes, 1999; Randall and McEwen, 2000).

Due to all these possible variations in context and opinion it is difficult to come up with a universal definition of a 'rehabilitation goal' that suits all clinical work. Wade (1998), however, writing for an interprofessional audience, offered one alternative, defining a 'goal' as: 'A future state that is desired and/or expected. The state might refer to relative changes or to an absolute achievement. It might refer to matters affecting the patient, the patient's environment, the family or any other party. It is a generic term with no implications about time frame or level' (Wade, 1998, p. 273).

The key point here, however, is that although it is arguable that all human behaviour is goal directed, and that rehabilitation cannot therefore occur without having goals of some kind, it is not true that all goals are 'rehabilitation goals' in the sense usually intended by rehabilitation teams. Rehabilitation goals are actively selected, intentionally created, have a purpose and ideally are shared by the people participating in the activities and interventions designed to address the consequences of acquired disability.

What is 'goal setting' and 'goal planning'?

In clinical rehabilitation, Wade (1998) has suggested that the terms 'goal setting' and 'goal planning' can be considered synonymous, defining them as: 'The process of agreeing on goals, this agreement usually being between the patient and all other interested parties' (Wade, 1998, p. 273). Similarly, Playford et al. (2000) have suggested that goal setting is: 'The process of agreeing on a desirable and achievable future state'. Nevertheless, in rehabilitation both goal setting and goal planning usually refer to a relationship between an individual patient and an individual or group of health professionals plus any other involved individuals such as family members. Goal setting should involve some degree of communication about the hopes, expectations, and intentions of all people involved in a single episode of rehabilitation, and a negotiation of the direction in which rehabilitation should head.

Application of goal planning to rehabilitation

As shown in Table 4.2, multiple approaches to goal setting in rehabilitation exist. These approaches can differ in terms of a number of factors such as the professional group (or groups) intended to use the approach, the intended patient population for the approach, the process by which goals are selected or negotiated, the recommended characteristics of the actual goals set (e.g. whether or not they should be measureable, activity related, realistic or ambitious and so on), the intended reason for having goals for rehabilitation or participating in goal setting, and the way the goals are subsequently used in the clinical environments. However, there are a few features that are common to many standard approaches to goal setting in rehabilitation, typically involving the following:

- finding out about the perspectives of the patient (and family) regarding their expected and/or desired outcomes from rehabilitation;
- finding out from the patient (and family) information about the context of their life outside of rehabilitation including their personal values, priorities, strengths, roles, relationships, and usual living environments (considering both physical and social factors);
- communicating information to the patient (and family) regarding clinical perspectives on the causes of their impairments and activity limitations, clinical factors influencing their prognosis for recovery, and the likely effectiveness of rehabilitation options;
- identifying long-term goals with patients and their family;
- identifying short-term (and sometimes medium-term) goals with patients and their family;
- identification of the actions (or 'tasks') required to achieve the goals, and the assignment of roles and responsibilities to the various people involved in undertaking these actions;
- specification of time frames for achievement or re-evaluation of goals;
- documentation of all long-term goals, medium-term goals, short-term goals, tasks, assigned responsibilities and time frames using a standardized template. (See Figure 4.3 for an example of a basic template.)

These activities can be carried out as part of a formal meeting with the patient, their family and relevant members of the clinical team. If a formal meeting is planned then the patient, their family and clinical staff should all be adequately prepared for this meeting (see also Chapter 3). Preparation of the patient and their family should involve providing education about the rehabilitation process and the role of goal setting within it, giving them sufficient time to consider what they would like to raise for discussion at the meeting.

Consideration ought to be given to *when* the initial goal-planning meeting is best held with patients and their families. If formal goal planning is delayed for too long, decisions about clinical interventions may have already been made and therapies implemented before goals are even set, making the whole goal-planning process far

GOAL PLANNING FORM

Patient ID

Name

Address

Long-term goals:

Date	Short-term goal	Tasks	Who/When	Evaluation
	1.			
	2.			
	3.			
	4.			
	5.			

Figure 4.3 Basic template for documentation of interprofessional goal planning.

less relevant. If goal planning is undertaken too quickly however, insufficient time may have been spent on building a rapport with the patient and their family, learning about their priorities and usual social context, before goals are set. There are no firm rules about when is best to set initial goals for rehabilitation, but one guideline might be that the longer and more complex the anticipated rehabilitation programme, the more time should be spent on building a working relationship with the patient and their family before confirming the goals of rehabilitation. In these types of service, pushing patients to set goals for therapy within their first interactions with clinicians, before they have had time to consider the implication of their newly acquired disability, may well be premature and result in superficial, tokenistic goals, rather than goals that reflect their personal context and world view.

Setting long-term goals

Prior to setting short-term goals and assigning clinical tasks, it is usually a good idea to establish the patient's long-term goals. In rehabilitation the phrase 'long-term goal' is sometimes used just to refer to any goal that is to be achieved at a more distant point in time (e.g. after discharge from a service or after a set period such as 4 or more weeks), with 'short-term goals' being the 'steps' required to make progress towards this 'long-term goal' (e.g. to be achieved after periods of 2 weeks or less). However, 'long-terms goals' can often be qualitatively different from 'short-term goals' as well. For example the phrase 'long-term goals' can at times be used to refer to: (1) goals that emphasize the direction the patient wishes to take with their life, (2) goals that are stated by the patient without reinterpretation or negotiation by the rehabilitation team, or (3) goals that are grouped under the ICF category of 'participation'.

Long-term goals can be identified by simply asking patients questions such as 'where do you see yourself in 6 months' time?' or 'what do you hope to eventually achieve from rehabilitation?' If this open-ended approach is unsuccessful then prompts under headings such as 'family', 'work', 'leisure', 'community activities', 'social relationships' and 'friends' may provide the starting points for discussion about these goals. In some situations (for example if the client has cognitive problems) this discussion will benefit from input from members of their family.

Alternatively, long-term goals can be established by using some method for identifying a patient's life goals. Life goals have been defined as 'the desired states that people seek to obtain, maintain or avoid' (Nair, 2003). Although a number of tools are available to evaluate life goals (Conrad et al., 2010; Nair, 2003), there is one tool designed specifically for the purpose of facilitating meaningful goal planning in rehabilitation settings and this is the Rivermead Life Goals Questionnaire (RLGQ). A copy of this questionnaire has been reproduced in Figure 4.4.

One important point regarding the RLGQ is that although 'scores' can be generated from its items, it has in no way been promoted as an outcome measure. This is because it is impossible to say whether changes in scores on individual RLGQ items represent improvements or deterioration in health outcomes. Also of note, apart from the original development work that went into the RLGQ (McGrath and Adams, 1999),

Various aspects and areas of life are given below. I would like you to tell me how important each is to you. Please rate the importance of each:

0 = of no importance,

1 = of some importance,

2 = of great importance, and

3 = of extreme importance.

	Domain	Rating	Comments
1	My residential and domestic arrangements (where I live and who with) are	0 1 2 3	
2	My ability to manage my personal care (dressing, toilet, washing) is	0 1 2 3	
3	My leisure, hobbies and interests including pets are	0 1 2 3	
4	My work, paid or unpaid is	0 1 2 3	
5	My relationship with my partner (or my wish to have one)	0 1 2 3	
6	My family life (including with those not living at home) is	0 1 2 3	
7	My contacts with friends, neighbours and acquaintances are	0 1 2 3	
8	My religion or life philosophy is	0 1 2 3	
9	My financial status is	0 1 2 3	

Figure 4.4   Rivermead Life Goals Questionnaire. (Courtesy of Rivermead Rehabilitation Centre, Abingdon Road, Oxford, UK.)

which suggested that RLGQ scores had adequate test–retest reliability, very little other research has been conducted on the psychometric properties of this assessment tool or to develop it further.

Nevertheless, scores resulting from application of the RLGQ can be useful and, at times, surprising: patients might indicate that they have no interest whatsoever in managing their personal cares but rather would like to focus more on abilities that could return them most quickly to leisure activities that they previously enjoyed; people who otherwise appear to be in a stable, long-term relationships might indicate that in fact the strength of their personal relationships with a spouse matters to them very little at all. Thus, the RLGQ helps clinicians (who are otherwise, frankly, strangers in their patients' lives) avoid making assumptions about individual patients based on superficial appearances, clinical experiences or on the clinician's own values and priorities. The RLGQ can also be a very useful tool for 'breaking the ice' with patients, facilitating a way into discussion of things other than the patient's immediate health problems when goal setting.

Setting short-term goals

Short-term goals are generally set by the rehabilitation team in negotiation with the patient. Short-term goals may start as objectives for rehabilitation identified by patients or may be simply recommended by a health professional as a necessary step towards achieving the patient's long-term goal. Regardless, short-term goals are usually converted into some type of standardized format according to the rehabilitation team's preferences, usually to make the goal more objective or to fit within what the clinicians believe they can provide. Most short-term goals are set at the ICF level of 'activity'. For example, goals focusing on a patient's ability to walk to the bus stop, manage basic financial transactions and tolerate light physical activity might be the subject of short-terms goals leading on to a long-term goal of returning to work.

Time frames are universally recommended for short-term goals, indicating a point at which the achievement, non-achievement or progress towards the goal is to be evaluated. In an interprofessional context, individual health professionals may have more or less responsibility than their colleagues to help patients achieve some specific short-term goals – although most goals are usually intended as 'team' goals, the achievement of which is part of the overall rehabilitation plan. Common approaches to standardizing short-term goals include use of the 'SMART' acronym, Randall and McEwen's (2000) 'who, what, how well, by when' method, and Goal Attainment Scaling (GAS).

'SMART' goals

One commonly promoted approach to standardization of short-term goals is the use of the 'SMART' acronym. To confuse matters, however, there is no single, agreed interpretation regarding what this acronym stands for (Wade, 2009). Schut and Stam (1994), in the earliest health science publication to mention SMART goals, stated that the SMART acronym referred to goals that were Specific, Motivating, Attainable, Rational and Timed (Schut and Stam, 1994). Alternatively, McLellan (1997) used this acronym to emphasize that goals should be Specific, Measurable, Activity-related, Realistic and Time-specific, whereas Barnes and Ward (2000) preferred Specific, Measurable, Achievable, Relevant and Time-limited. Other version of the SMART acronym also exist (Marsland and Bowman, 2010; Mastos et al., 2007; Monaghan et al., 2005; Wilson, 2008).

Rubin (2002) suggested that the SMART approach to goal planning originated as a way to quickly communicate decades of research from industrial organizational psychology, but that over time, as people attempted to fit SMART goals into different contexts, the acronym drifted away from its original meaning and from the research on which it was based. This may explain in part the differences in the recommended qualities of goals resulting from the SMART approach: these various interpretations may be based more on clinical opinion rather than high-quality research. For instance, from a research perspective there is no consistent evidence that goals that are 'realistic' or 'achievable' result in better health outcomes for rehabilitation patients than goals that are highly ambitious or difficult to achieve (Levack et al., 2006c). In fact, research from the field of industrial organizational psychology has suggested that challenging short-term goals, which might be difficult to achieve, tend to result in higher levels of performance on work tasks than goals that are easily achievable (Locke and Latham, 2002).

Randall and McEwen's 'who, what, how well, by when' method

One other problem with SMART goals is that the acronym gives little guidance regarding how to actually make a goal 'specific' or 'measurable' and so on. Randall and McEwen's (2000) approach to documentation of goals provides a similar format to that of the SMART acronym, but with clearer guidelines around how to actually document a goal. Randall and McEwen (2000) recommended that all documented goals should include information to answer the following five questions: who will do what, under what conditions, how well and by when? According to these authors, the 'Who?' of the goal should always be the patient. The question 'Will do what?' refers to the functional activity that the patient will be to be able to carry out on completion of therapy. The question 'Under what conditions?' provides a prompt to therapists to consider the environmental context under which the activity is to be performed (for example, if the subject of goal is 'to be able to dress oneself', the condition under which this goal is to be performed might include reference to the use of Velcro fasteners, reaching tools or memory aids). Information about 'How well?' the goal is to be completed refers to the quality of performance (e.g. the number of attempts required to complete the task), the amount of additional assistance (e.g. whether the activity is to be complete independently, with verbal prompts or with minimal physical assistance etc), or the speed for completion of the task (e.g. within 10 minutes). Finally, the question 'By when?' indicates the need to include a time frame by when achievement or non-achievement of the goals is to be evaluated. Thus, following Randall and McEwen's method, a documented short-term goal might read something like: 'That Mary will dress her bottom half, with use of chair for balance and assistance of one person to put on her shoes and socks, within 2 weeks.'

Goal Attainment Scaling (GAS) goals

One other approach to setting short-term goals is the use of Goal Attainment Scaling (GAS). Originally developed by Kiresuk and Sherman (1968), GAS was initially designed to evaluate patient outcomes in mental health services. Because of this emphasis on using goals for outcome measurement, Kiresuk and Sherman (1968) were explicit that neither the patient nor the treating clinicians should be involved in either the selection of goals or the evaluation of goal attainment. Instead, their method involved a third party (e.g. a non-treating clinician) developing the GAS scale for individual patients and scoring the patients against those scales on completion of therapy.

Of course, nowadays the potential therapeutic effects of goal setting are valued far more highly, and the distinction between using goals for improving patient outcomes versus using goals for measuring patient outcomes has become far less clear cut.

Typically, the treating clinician, the patient, and (at times) their family are involved in the process of selection of goals and in the development of individualized GAS scales. GAS usually involves selecting one or more goals for therapy, and, for each goal, describing an ordinal scale of five favourable to unfavourable outcomes. The mid-point on this scale of possible outcomes should be set as the *most expected* outcome of treatment and given the score '0', with the scores '+2' and '+1' being assigned to potential outcomes that were better than expected and '–2' and '–1' being assigned to those that were worse than expected (Kiresuk and Sherman, 1968). Proponents of this method argue that GAS scores offer a way of quantifying the level of achievement of goals, and thus a means of evaluating the effectiveness of the rehabilitation programme.

For a detailed description on how to develop GAS goals, how to score them and how to apply them to rehabilitation, readers are advised to consider guidelines provided by Turner-Stokes (2009). One of Turner-Stokes' (2009) recommendations has been that in clinical work (as opposed to research) it is sufficient to use standardized terminology for all but the '0' score. This involves using the phrases 'greatly exceeded expected outcome', 'slightly exceeded expected outcome', 'not quite achieved expected outcome', and 'nowhere near the expected outcome' for the scores '+2', '+1', '–1' and '–2' respectively. (Time is still required to carefully operationalize what is the 'expected outcome', which is of course the '0' score on the GAS scale, and for this task Turner-Stokes again refers to the SMART acronym as a guide.) This approach significantly reduces the amount of time required for developing all of the levels on the GAS scale, while still producing (according to Turner-Stokes) an individualized outcome measure related to the personal goals of each patients. (See Table 4.3 for a comparison of the original and abbreviated approaches.)

Table 4.3 Standard versus individualized methods for establishing Goal Attainment Scaling (GAS) levels.

GAS score	Individual scale items	Standardized scale items
+2	That John will be able to walk up and down a flight of 12 steps six times in 2 minutes without use of a walking stick	Greatly exceed expected outcome
+1	That John will be able to walk up a flight of 12 steps independently without use of a walking stick	Slightly exceeded expected outcome
0	That John will be able to walk up a flight of 12 steps independently with aid of a walking stick	That John will be able to walk up a flight of stairs independently with aid of a walking stick
–1	That John will be able to walk up a flight of 12 steps with assistance of one person and a walking stick	Not quite achieved expected outcome
–2	That John will not be able to walk up a flight of 12 steps even with maximal assistance	Nowhere near the expected outcome

Considerations for goal planning

Purposes of goal planning

Although research has yet to provide clear and consistent evidence regarding the best approach to goal setting in rehabilitation (Levack et al., 2006c), it seems almost certainly true that no single approach to goal setting is going to be appropriate for all clinical environments or all individual patients. Approaches to goal planning need to be tailored to meet the individual needs of each rehabilitation service and each patient population. As alluded to above, goal setting has been attributed with many purposes (Levack et al., 2006a, 2006b). Purposes (or reasons) for valuing, prioritizing and undertaking goal planning have included the following beliefs:

- That goal setting might ultimately improve patient outcomes by:
  - improving a patient's motivation to engage in therapeutic activities;
  - improving clinical teamwork;
  - enhancing the working relationship between patients, families and health professionals;
  - assisting patients (and their family) to psychologically adapt to the consequences of disability (through discussion of what the future might bring, and priorities for that future);
  - enhancing the specificity of training of therapy (e.g. focusing therapy for an individual on performance of a specific functional ability and specific environmental context relevant to that individual's daily life);
- that goal setting might enhance patient autonomy;
- that the degree of goal attainment is a useful measure of health outcome;
- that goal setting is a contractual or legislative requirement of service delivery.

It might seem possible or desirable to have one approach to goal planning that can achieve all of these outcomes, however, on closer investigation it becomes apparent that some reasons for undertaking goal setting can conflict with others. For instance, if goals are going to be used primarily as a way of evaluating health outcomes, with perhaps a third-party payer requiring goal attainment to be reported for auditing or contractual purposes, then clinicians are going to be far less inclined to use goal setting for the purpose of enhancing patient self-determination – particularly if patients wish to pursue goals that the therapists believe are unlikely to be achieved. Similarly, ambitious goals designed to enhance motivation (see below) may conflict with goal setting for the purpose of outcome evaluation. Thus, when deciding on a shared approach to goal planning, rehabilitation teams are advised to spend time discussing their beliefs around reasons for using goal planning in their service. A shared understanding of the purpose of goals in rehabilitation is beneficial for developing an agreed, standardized approach to rehabilitation planning for patients.

Disrupted life goals

Impairments and disability can have a direct impact on an individual's future, presenting barriers to past objectives and ambitions, removing opportunities that might previously have existed, but also creating new prospects. Changes in future opportunities can occur suddenly for some people (e.g. in the event of serious accidents) or slowly (e.g. in the case of degenerative or long-term conditions). Chronic ill health and disability can also make people re-evaluate who they are and what their life means and this topic will be discussed again in Chapter 6. However, as just one example of this, in a meta-synthesis of qualitative research, Levack and colleagues (2010) examined the lived experience of recovery and outcome following traumatic brain injury. Among the findings from this review was the reported experience of loss and reconstruction of self-identity and personhood. In other words, following traumatic brain injury, not only do people have to deal with (and attempt to recover from) loss of physical and cognitive abilities, loss of social roles and loss of social networks – they also have to deal with changes in their perceptions of who they are as people. These sorts of experiences can produce intense existential crises for some people; ones which they often have to face alone.

Although some of the experience of loss of self-identity and personhood for people with traumatic brain injury is no doubt related to damage to specific areas of the brain, changes in self-identity have also been reported in qualitative research involving people with other conditions such as stroke (Salter et al., 2008) and spinal cord injury (Hammell, 2007). Changes in self-identity following injury and illness appears, at least in part, to be related to changes in life roles, life opportunities and how individuals are treated as people by others.

Furthermore, as noted by Nair (2003), research into life goals has suggested that there may be some relationship between having 'a high sense of well being [and] … recognition of life goals, commitment to life goals, perception of progress toward life goal, and sense of achievement of life goals' (Nair, 2003, p. 194). For instance, Nair and Wade (2003) reported that people with neurological disabilities who were more depressed tended to have fewer life goals that they valued as extremely important than those who were not depressed. Similarly, Conrad et al. (2010) undertook a study to examine the relationship between life goals and subjective well-being in a population of adults receiving rehabilitation for brain injury. Conrad and colleagues (2010) used the 'Life Goals Questionnaire' to assess the importance, attainability and perception of success with life goals. The Life Goals Questionnaire is a theoretically driven assessment tool, which consists of 24 items that evaluates life goals in six main areas: intimacy, affiliation (time spent with others), altruism, power (high social status), achievement (improving skills) and variation (excitement in life). Conrad et al. (2010) found that the most important life goal categories for people participating in rehabilitation were in the intimacy, achievement and altruism domains. The best predictor of subjective well-being, according to Conrad et al. (2010), was success in 'achievement' life goals (i.e. patients who felt they made continuing gains in skills and abilities were more likely to experience high subjective well-being than those who were not), but also strongly associated with high subjective well-being was the discrepancy between a patient's rating of 'importance' in the intimacy domain and their rating of 'success' in that domain. In particular, patients who highly valued intimacy life goals, but who believed they had not been successful in this area of their life following disability, were more likely to experience poorer subjective well-being.

The process of goal planning can therefore have some impact, either directly or indirectly, on assisting patients to reconnect with or reconstruct their life goals following injury or illness. One approach, developed to assist people with 'reinventing' themselves after acquired disability is called 'Identity Oriented Goal Mapping' (Ylvisaker and Feeney, 2000; Ylvisaker et al., 2008). In this approach to goal setting, patients are first asked to identify a 'hero' figure in their lives – a person they admire and wish to be more like. The process of identity oriented goal mapping then continues on with discussions between the clinicians and patient regarding the feelings, values and characteristics of that hero figure, leading onto identification of what actions could be pursued to become more like that idealized self. These actions then inform the development of long-term and short-term goals of therapy. The assumption here is that goals resulting from such an approach are more meaningful, more personal and therefore more motivating for individual patients who are engaging in rehabilitation programmes.

Impairments of goal pursuit

Of course, even when people have a clear understanding of what kind of person they want to be and what kind of goals they want to pursue, they may not always have the skills to act on those objectives. The capacity to change or maintain one's behaviour in order to advance toward a desired goal is a large part of what has been called 'self-regulation'. Importantly, some forms of injury and illness (such as mental health conditions or brain injury) can directly affect a person's capacity for self-regulation.

One approach to retraining self-regulation skills has been proposed by Levine et al. (2000). Derived from a theory of 'goal neglect', Levine et al. (2000) developed a protocol for making the steps of self-regulation explicit in order to share them, as a taught activity, with people who had executive functioning problems resulting from traumatic brain injury. They called this approach 'Goal Management Training' (GMT). In a randomized controlled trial involving 30 people with traumatic brain injury, Levine et al. (2000) found that GMT resulted in significantly greater improvements on everyday paper-and-pencil tasks when compared with a control group receiving motor skills training. Although cautious in their conclusions Levine and colleagues (2000) suggested that goal management skills learnt through GMT may be generalizable to other everyday activities that are not specifically the focus of an intervention.

Not all problems with goal pursuit are necessarily the result of impairments however. Some people who enter healthcare services might never have had terribly sophisticated self-regulation skills prior to injury or illness. Furthermore, a well-meaning but paternalistic rehabilitation service can even act to impede the development of self-regulation skills in patients. In an article on self-regulation in paediatric rehabilitation, Ylvisaker and Feeney (2002) noted that '… the near total control that well-meaning staff and parents often exercise over children with brain injury with the goal of facilitating rehabilitation and self-regulation may have an effect opposite the intended effect' (Ylvisaker and Feeney, 2002, p. 60). The authors' point was that in order for children to learn skills in self-regulation, they need opportunities to practise such skills. This would involve opportunities to participate in goal setting, opportunities to initiate activities (rather than just following the therapist's lead in activities) and opportunities to monitor and evaluate their own progress. Just as 'doing for' people with physical impairments prevents opportunities to regain independent physical abilities (e.g. washing, dressing, toileting), 'thinking for' people with executive functioning impairments prevents opportunities to regain abilities in self-regulation (e.g. decision making, planning, risk evaluation). No doubt there are lessons to be learnt here for adult rehabilitation and chronic condition management as well.

4.4 Interventions

Classification of rehabilitation interventions

Rehabilitation involves a considerable range of different interventions. Several attempts have been made to develop a classification system to describe these interventions (Abraham and Michie, 2008; DeJong et al., 2004; Livneh, 1989; Scofield et al., 1980; Sigelman et al., 1979; Wade, 2005; Whiteneck et al., 2009), but no one taxonomy appears to have been universally accepted across all fields of rehabilitation.

What is apparent is that the classification of rehabilitation interventions is complex. There are a number of reasons for this. First, almost all rehabilitation interventions are experience based and relationship based (Hart, 2009). In other words, rehabilitation interventions depend not only on what health professionals *do*, but also on how they *engage* with patients and the significant other people in their lives and, reciprocally, how patients engage with them. Interventions can involve not only modalities to influence health and function but also can be directed toward changing how patients think about their disability, their motivation, their capacity for achieving goals (i.e. their self-efficacy) and the way they undertake therapeutic activities.

Second, most rehabilitation interventions involve a number of interacting components. For example, an occupational therapist may use a simple baking activity to help an older adult regain skills in activities of daily living after a stroke. However, the activity itself may include strengthening of weak muscles in a hemiplegic arm and leg (lifting and using kitchen utensils; bending and reaching), retraining of balance (moving around the kitchen), cardiovascular exercise conditioning and fatigue management, training in the use of assistive technology (mobility aids and adapted kitchen implements) and cognitive retraining (following a recipe; safe use of an oven). Concurrently, the occupational therapist may also use the same therapy session as an opportunity to provide some education for the older adult on the nature of stroke and how to adjust for deficits in function on return home, as well as providing general emotional counselling and support. Furthermore, the occupational therapist may conduct their treatment as a combined session with another member of their rehabilitation team (e.g. the speech language therapist or physiotherapist), taking the opportunity to work collaboratively to address a patient's various functional limitations.

Third, rehabilitation interventions involve a considerable degree of creativity and flexibility when tailoring treatments to meet the individual needs of patients. Rehabilitation is a problem-focused intervention. The specific nature of therapeutic tasks are continually adapted by rehabilitation professionals depending not only on the particular spectrum of impairments that a patient might present with, but also on the specific goals of rehabilitation for that individual, the environmental context under which a patient is performing targeted activities, and on the personality and personal interests of the patient. Rehabilitation interventions can also be provided individually or in groups, and in different clinical settings such as a rehabilitation gym or in 'real world' environments in the community, with different benefits and disadvantages to each approach.

One early approach to classification of rehabilitation interventions proposed by Livneh (1989) involved consideration of three variables: (1) the environmental context of the rehabilitation programme, (2) the adjustment domain, and (3) the focus (or subject) of the interventions. Livneh (1989) suggested that each of these variables could be dichotomized. The environmental context of rehabilitation, according to Livneh (1989), could either be 'the community' or 'the workplace', the adjustment domain was categorized as either being 'physical' or 'psychosocial', and the intervention itself could either focus on changing 'the environment' or 'the patient'. Livneh's (1989) system thus resulted in the classification of eight types of rehabilitation intervention (i.e. eight possible combinations of these three pairs of variables). So, for instance, providing a patient with exercises to improve his or her ability to dress independently would be an example of a community-based physical intervention, targeting the patient to make behavioural changes or functional gains. Whereas, providing an employer with education about traumatic brain injury in order to support a person to gain work after injury, would be an example of a work-based psychosocial intervention aimed at achieving a positive employment outcome through changing the work environment rather than changing anything specifically about the individual with brain injury. Although suitable for many rehabilitation situations, Livneh's (1989) system does, however, have some obvious gaps. Rehabilitation does not occur in only two locations for instance (rehabilitation in educational settings is one clear omission) and a vast number of different types of interventions could still be listed under each of Livneh's (1989) eight categories.

Livneh's (1989) classification could be extended if a distinction were made between interventions that focus on *recovery* of body structure or body function versus those interventions that seek to address disability through *compensation* for impairments or activity limitations. Examples of recovery of body structure and body function would include, for example, a person with cardiac disease exercising to regain the cardiovascular fitness required to carry and hang washing on a line that is at the bottom of their garden. A compensation intervention would involve moving the washing line nearer so that the individual no longer requires a higher level of cardiovascular fitness to be independent with hanging out the washing. Although Livneh's (1989) classification could distinguish between these two interventions on the basis of the intervention foci (the person versus the environment), this is not the case for all interventions that target recovery versus compensation strategies. A person with a hemiplegic arm for instance could learn to dress independently by either regaining muscle strength, range of movement and dexterity in their weaker limb (recovery), or could gain independence simply by learning to dress entirely with the use of their unimpaired arm (compensation).

Although some have argued that interventions that focus on recovery are superior to those that focus on compensation (Levine et al., 2009), the risk of such a perspective is to overemphasize the importance of addressing impairments of body structure and body function when, as is described in Chapter 2, not all improvements in body structure and function have a direct correlation with improvements at the level of activity and social participation. Furthermore, people with disabilities themselves are not always as concerned about impairments (such as the 'quality' of their movement) as are their health professionals, provided that they can go where they want to go and do what they want to do.

More comprehensive approaches to categorization of rehabilitation interventions have arisen from research involving prospective observational studies methods, also known as 'practice-based evidence', for various health conditions (DeJong et al., 2004, 2009; Whiteneck et al., 2009). These studies have each involved the development of taxonomies of rehabilitation interventions, specific to particular area of clinical practice. These taxonomies, however, highlight further how complicated rehabilitation interventions can be. For instance, just the descriptions of the taxonomies of interventions for physical therapy, occupational therapy, recreational therapy, speech therapy, psychology, social work and nursing in the prospective observational study of rehabilitation for spinal cord injury filled an entire issue of a rehabilitation journal (Whiteneck et al., 2009).

Rehabilitation interventions should thus be considered multidimensional, interactive, experiential, comprehensive and flexible. Selection and prioritization of rehabilitation interventions should flow from the patient assessment and goal-setting processes if a person-centred approach to rehabilitation is to be undertaken. An evidence-based approach to treatment selection should always be considered in the design of any rehabilitation plan, but because of the individual nature of disability and rehabilitation goals, rehabilitation professionals need to be open to exploring new avenues for intervention and seek creative solutions to problems with activity limitation and participation restrictions. These solutions may involve treatments to address impairments of body structure and function, but equally may involve interventions to address environmental barriers to function or even to address personal factors that may interfere with patients achieving their life goals.

Motivation and adherence

The success of most (if not all) rehabilitation interventions is entirely dependent on the commitment and engagement of the people receiving the service. Adaptive equipment cannot facilitate higher levels of community integration if left in a cupboard. Therapists' levels of knowledge and skill in neuromuscular physiology and movement training are irrelevant if the person they are working with does not want to undertake exercises (which may be difficult, tedious, or uncomfortable to perform). Therefore, patient motivation and adherence is central to the notion of effective rehabilitation.

Maclean and Pound (2000) conducted a critical appraisal of literature on the concept of patient motivation in physical rehabilitation. In this review Maclean and Pound (2000) classified publications into three broad groups: (1) those that presented patient motivation as an internal personality trait, (2) those that presented patient motivation as a behavioural response to social and environmental factors, and (3) those that viewed motivation as an interaction between both internal personality traits and social/environmental factors.

If viewing patient motivation from the first of these perspectives, clinicians might consider patients as coming to rehabilitation with a fixed degree of internal motivation (ranging from very high to very low). They might consider those with low motivation as being less suitable for rehabilitation (maybe referring to them as an 'inappropriate' admissions decision). They might view those with high motivation as ideal candidates for rehabilitation, and consequentially spend more time with them. Importantly, if patient motivation is viewed primarily as a product of internal personality traits, clinicians are likely to view motivation as something that they cannot influence to any great extent. In fact, Maclean and colleagues have provided additional evidence that clinicians do indeed think along these lines at times. In one study exploring the beliefs of health professionals regarding patient motivation in stroke rehabilitation, Maclean et al. (2002) reported that clinicians were aware they tended to treat patients differently based on how motivated or unmotivated they appeared – preferring to interact more with patients who presented as motivated. The clinicians also described giving less encouragement to apparently 'unmotivated' adults over 75 years than equally unmotivated 50 years olds – so these judgements appeared somewhat age related (or, more accurately, ageist).

Viewing patient motivation as a behavioural response to social and environmental factors, however, is a different story. From this perspective clinicians and the health service as a whole can be viewed as part of the patient's social world, and therefore can be viewed as directly influencing their level of motivation to engage in rehabilitation activities. For example, manipulating variables associated with goal setting should, following this line of thinking, directly influence patient motivation. However, *which* goal-setting variables most influence changes in patient motivation is a question worthy of consideration.

In fact, there appears to be a least three possible ways that clinicians conceptualize the relationship between goal setting, interventions and patient motivation. The first explanation is that patients may become more motivated when they become aware of making tangible progress towards a goal or when a goal is achieved (Maclean et al., 2002; Schut and Stam, 1994). In other words, after attaining goals or progress towards a goal, patients are inspired to try harder with future rehabilitation activities.

This explanation fits with Bandura's Social Cognitive Theory in that experiencing success with progress toward one rehabilitation goal (even if only a small step on the pathway of recovery) could conceivably result in 'enactive attainment' (Bandura,

1997). Enactive attainment is the positive experience of mastery resulting from successful completion of an activity or pursuit, and is one of Bandura's four factors influencing a person's belief in their ability to attain goals (also called their 'self-efficacy').[1]

As one example of this from a clinical setting, Dixon (2007) conducted a qualitative study of goal setting in neurological rehabilitation where it was reported that the 'completion of goals help[ed] patients to recognize explicitly what they [were] achieving' (Dixon, 2007, p. 235), with Dixon linking this finding with patients becoming more motivated to continue with their rehabilitation.

Associated with this first explanation is a belief that goals can have the reverse effect and be de-motivating if patients fail to make progress. Some authors have suggested that lack of goal attainment may make patients 'despondent' (Schut and Stam, 1994). In the case of rehabilitation for people with chronic pain, Tripp (1999) advised that: 'Any goals or aims that are identified must be realistic and achievable, as setting unrealistic goals is doomed to end in failure, causing further reinforcement of the sense of hopelessness' (Tripp, 1999, p. 121). However, it is important to recognize that the application of these theories to goal setting in clinical rehabilitation is almost entirely opinion based, with little empirical evidence underpinning them (Levack et al., 2006c). It is questionable for instance whether goal attainment is always perceived as a positive and rewarding experience by patients, for example: the process of achieving the goal might require exertion and even pain, or it may be that the goals are considered so small that they are perceived by the patient to be patronizing or irrelevant.

The second explanation of the relationship between goal planning and motivation is that patients become motivated to pursue rehabilitation when the goals of therapy are viewed as being personally relevant (Maclean et al., 2002; Nair, 2003; Wade, 1999a). This theory relates motivation to life-goal hierarchies. In other words, the more personally meaningful a rehabilitation goal is to a patient, the more inclined they will be to participate in activities that appear to lead towards it. Following this approach to patient motivation, clinicians need to begin by first identifying the patient's 'life goals' before ensuring that all goals set by the rehabilitation team are explicitly aligned with these (Wade, 1999b; Nair, 2003).

The third explanation is that goals can *directly* influence a person's level of effort, persistence and attention to therapeutic tasks, contributing to their self-regulation during rehabilitation. In other words, people *strive* towards goals. Just having goals creates a point of focus for work. From this perspective, goals do not even need to be achieved (or achievable) before they can exert an influence on behaviour. As mentioned earlier, one core finding from the Locke and Latham's (2002) goal theory is that specific, difficult goals produce higher levels of effort and performance when

---

[1] The other three factor that Bandura (1997) proposed influence self-efficacy are: 'modelling', when people learn vicariously by watching their peers, 'social persuasion', which occurs when other people try to convince an individual that they are capable of achieving success, and 'physiological factors', which refers to factors such as increased heart rate and arousal associated with higher level of physical or psychological stress.

compared with non-specific or specific, easy goals, although this effect is moderated by a number of factors such as goal commitment, self-efficacy and task complexity.

What these ideas suggest is that there are many factors, like goal setting, that can contribute to facilitating treatment adherence. It is certainly more complex than just educating patients or providing them with more information about what they should or should not be doing. Taking the time to find out what underlies peoples' motivation and their expectations of treatment can be very informative when planning the right rehabilitation intervention with the patient. For example, in a research study of people with myocardial infarctions, patients were more likely to attend the cardiac rehabilitation exercise sessions and ultimately return to work if their beliefs about heart disease and their expectations of the exercise sessions 'matched' with what the cardiac rehabilitation was set up to achieve (Petrie et al., 2002). In other words those patients who believed their heart attack was the result of stress and also believed exercise would cause further stress to their hearts were less likely to attend the sessions; if they had found their work stressful it did not make sense to try to return to work, as this work stress was what had caused the heart attack in the first place. Equally if smoking and drinking were things they did to relieve their stress then it did not make sense to these people to give these things up. In any rehabilitation setting, taking time to elucidate patients' common sense beliefs about the cause of their condition and their expectations of recovery, and if need be helping them towards a more appropriate match, is a crucial part of the rehabilitation planning process.

4.5   Evaluation

The rehabilitation cycle finishes with evaluation of the patient's health outcomes. This might include assessment of the degree to which a patient has achieved their individual goals or through use of a standardized outcome measure. On the basis of this evaluation, it can be then be decided whether the patient should be discharged from the rehabilitation service, should continue with current intervention for a bit longer, or whether a new course of action with different goals and different interventions is required.

Chapter 5 provides a comprehensive overview of the considerations that are required when selecting and using outcome measures in rehabilitation. However, some thought should be given here to the use of goal attainment for evaluating the effectiveness of completed interventions and hence how they relate to evaluation as part of the rehabilitation process. Provided that rehabilitation goals have been written relatively objectively, goal attainment can be evaluated on the basis of a simple decision whether the goal has been completed or not. Alternatively, if using a structured process for evaluation of goal attainment, such as GAS (Turner-Stokes, 2009), a score can be derived to represent the degree of goal attainment.

These methods carry a certain amount of face validity. It *feels* appropriate to rehabilitation professionals to evaluate the success of their interventions on the basis of whether or not they achieved what they thought they would achieve with their patients. However, one problem with this method of evaluation is that it is always open to a degree of retrospective interpretation. If a goal is successfully reached, the health professional is likely to think that their chosen interventions were effective, but if a goal is not reached, then the health professional could *either* decide their interventions were not effective *or* that the goals were unrealistic to begin with.

Nevertheless, for individual patients (as opposed to populations of people), thinking about what goals were set and whether these were achieved provides one way of reflecting on an individual's progress and provides a useful framework for discussion of future plans for that individual's rehabilitation, discharge from one health service, or referral to another.

4.6 Discharge planning and transitions from hospital to community

So far in this chapter the rehabilitation process has been considered from the perspective of a single rehabilitation service. However, people with newly acquired disabilities frequently engage with multiple services. Patients can start off in an acute medical or surgical ward before being transferred to an inpatient rehabilitation facility, after which they may be transferred to a community-based rehabilitation service, which might see them in a residential setting, in their own home or elsewhere in the community. The co-ordination of rehabilitation during these periods of transition or discharge is very important and needs to be planned for. Unfortunately, these periods of transition are frequently difficult and stressful for people with newly acquired disabilities (Cott, 2007; Ellis-Hill et al., 2009; Turner et al., 2008). Further, poor management of hospital discharge carries with it the risk of people needing to be re-admitted (Scott, 2010). This poses a significant problem as in the UK, for instance, hospital re-admissions are increasing, with 11.5% of all unplanned admissions being due to re-admission within 28 days of a discharge from hospital (Blunt et al., 2010). Chapter 6 provides more detail regarding factors that make the process of transition between services or discharge from services more problematic, and strategies which can be used to improve this aspect of the rehabilitation process.

4.7 Conclusion

The rehabilitation process is a dynamic one that requires health professionals to actively engage with patients and their families in the planning and implementation of interventions. Rehabilitation is about providing opportunities and solving problems. Rehabilitation professionals need to be creative and flexible in their work. They need to develop robust plans for treatment or intervention, based on the needs and preferences of their patients, but be capable of adjusting these plans should initial strategies prove ineffective or as different goals for rehabilitation arise.

Additional resources

An online tutorial, *Goal Setting in Adult Neurology*, developed by Rachel Barnard for the Centre for Excellent in Teaching and Learning (CETL) is available at: http://www.cetl.org.uk/learning/Overview_of_the_goal_setting%20literature/player.html (accessed 16 March 2012).

Barnes, M. P. and Ward, A. B. (2000). *Textbook of Rehabilitation Medicine.* Oxford: Oxford University Press.

French, D., Vedhara, K., Kaptein, A.A. and Weinman, J. (Editors) (2010). *Health Psychology (2nd edn).* Oxford: BPS Blackwell. In particular the chapter by Horne, R. and Clatworthy, J., *Adherence to advice and treatment.*

References

Abraham, C. and Michie, S. (2008). A taxonomy of behaviour change techniques used in interventions. *Health Psychology, 27*(3), 379–387.

Åsenlöf, P. and Silijebäck, K. (2009). Goal priority questionnaire is moderately reproducible in people with persistent musculoskeletal pain. *Physical Therapy, 89,* 1226–1234.

Austin, J. T. and Vancouver, J. B. (1996). Goal constructs in psychology: structure, process and content. *Psychological Bulletin, 120*(3), 338–375.

Bandura, A. (1997). *Self-efficacy: The Exercise of Control.* New York: Freeman.

Barnes, M. P. and Ward, A. B. (2000). *Textbook of Rehabilitation Medicine.* Oxford: Oxford University Press.

Barnett, D. (1999). The rehabilitation nurse as educator. In: M. Smith. (Editor). *Rehabilitation in Adult Nursing Practice.* Edinburgh: Churchill Livingstone, pp. 53–76.

Blunt, I., Bardsley, M., and Dixon, J. (2010). *Trends in Emergency Admissions in England 2004–2009: Is Greater Efficiency Breeding Inefficiency?* London: The Nuffield Trust.

Bovend'Eerdt, T. J. H., Botell, R. E. and Wade, D. T. (2009). Writing SMART rehabilitation goals and achieving goal attainment scaling: a practical guide. *Clinical Rehabilitation, 23,* 352–361.

Clarke, S. P., Oades, L.G., Crowe, T. P. and Deane, F. P. (2006). Collaborative goal technology: theory and practice. *Psychiatric Rehabilitation Journal, 30*(2), 129–136.

Conrad, N., Doering, B. K., Rief, W. and Exner, C. (2010). Looking beyond the importance of life goals. The personal goal model of subjective well-being in neuropsychological rehabilitation. *Clinical Rehabilitation, 24,* 431–443.

Cott, C. A. (2007). Continuity, transition and participation: preparing clients for life in the community post-stroke. *Disability and Rehabilitation, 29*(20–21), 1566–1574.

DeJong, G., Horn, S. D., Gassaway, J., Slavin, M. D. and Dijkers, M. P. (2004). Toward a Taxonomy of Rehabilitation Interventions: using an inductive approach to examine the "black box" of rehabilitation. *Archives of Physical Medicine & Rehabilitation, 85*(4), 678–686.

DeJong, G., Hsieh, C., Gassaway, J., Horn, S. D., Smout, R. J. and Putman, K. (2009). Characterizing rehabilitation services for patients with knee and hip replacement in skilled nursing facilities and inpatient rehabilitation facilities. *Archives of Physical Medicine & Rehabilitation, 90,* 1269–1283.

Dixon, G. (2007). Perceptions of self-efficacy and rehabilitation among neurologically disabled adults. *Clinical Rehabilitation, 21,* 230–240.

Ellis-Hill, C., Robison, J., Wiles, R., McPherson, K., Hyndman, D. and Ashburn, A. (2009). Going home to get on with life: patients and carers experiences of being discharged from hospital following a stroke. *Disability and Rehabilitation*, *31*(2), 61–72.

Hammell, K. W. (2007). Quality of life after spinal cord injury: a meta-synthesis of qualitative findings. *Spinal Cord*, *45*(2), 124–139.

Hart, T. (2009). Treatment definition in complex rehabilitation interventions. *Neuropsychological Rehabilitation*, *19*(6), 824–840.

Kiresuk, T. and Sherman, R. (1968). Goal Attainment Scaling: a general method for evaluating community health programs. *Community Mental Health Journal*, *4*, 443–453.

Levack, W. M. M., Dean, S. G., Siegert, R. J. and McPherson, K. M. (2006a). Purposes and mechanisms of goal planning in rehabilitation: the need for a critical distinction. *Disability and Rehabilitation*, *28*(12), 741–749.

Levack, W. M. M., Dean, S.G., McPherson, K. M. and Siegert, R. J. (2006b). How clinicians talk about the application of goal planning to rehabilitation for people with brain injury – variable interpretations of value and purpose. *Brain Injury*, *20*(13–14), 1439–1449.

Levack, W. M. M., Taylor, K., Siegert, R. J., Dean, S. G., McPherson, K. M. and Weatherall, M. (2006c). Is goal planning in rehabilitation effective? A systematic review. *Clinical Rehabilitation*, *20*(9), 739–755.

Levack, W. M. M., Siegert, R. J., Dean, S. G. and McPherson, K. M. (2009). Goal planning for adults with acquired brain injury: how clinicians talk about involving family. *Brain Injury*, *23*(3), 192–202.

Levack, W. M. M., Kayes, N. M. and Fadyl, J. K. (2010). Experience of recovery and outcome following traumatic brain injury: a metasynthesis of qualitative research. *Disability and Rehabilitation*, *32*(12), 986–999.

Levine, B., Robertson, I. H., Clare, L., Carter, G., Hong, J., Wilson, B. A., Duncan, J. and Stuss, D. T. (2000). Rehabilitation of executive functioning: an experimental-clinical validation of goal management training. *Journal of the International Neuropsychological Society*, *6*(3), 299–312.

Levine, M., Kleim, J. A. and Wolf, S. L. (2009). What do motor 'recovery' and 'compensation' mean in patients following stroke? *Neurorehabilitation and Neural Repair*, *23*(4), 313–319.

Livneh, H. (1989). Rehabilitation intervention strategies: their integration and classification. *Journal of Rehabilitation*, *55*, 21–30.

Locke, E. A. and Latham, G. P. (2002). Building a practically useful theory of goal setting and task motivation: a 35-year odyssey. *American Psychologist*, *57*(9), 705–717.

Maclean, N. and Pound, P. (2000). A critical review of the concept of patient motivation in the literature on physical rehabilitation. *Social Science and Medicine*, *50*(4), 495–506.

Maclean, N., Pound, P., Wolfe, C. and Rudd, A. (2002). The concept of patient motivation: a qualitative analysis of stroke professionals' attitudes. *Stroke*, *33*(2), 444–450.

Marsland, E. and Bowman, J. (2010). An interactive education session and follow-up support as a strategy to improve clinicians' goal-writing skills: a randomized controlled trial. *Journal of Evaluation in Clinical Practice*, *16*, 3–13.

Mastos, M., Miller, K., Eliasson, A. C. and Imms, C. (2007). Goal-directed training: linking theories of treatment to clinical practice for improved functional activities in daily life. *Clinical Rehabilitation*, *21*, 47–55.

McGrath, J. R. and Adams, L. (1999). Patient-centred goal planning: a systemic psychological therapy? *Topics in Stroke Rehabilitation*, *6*(2), 43–50.

McGrath, J. R. and Davis, A.M. (1992). Rehabilitation: where are we going and how do we get there? *Clinical Rehabilitation*, *6*, 225–235.

McGrath, J. R., Marks, J. A. and Davis, A. M. (1995). Towards interdisciplinary rehabilitation: further developments at Rivermead Rehabiliation Centre. *Clinical Rehabilitation*, *9*, 320–326.

McLellan, D. L. (1997). Introduction to rehabilitation. In: B. A. Wilson and D. L. McLellan (Editors). *Rehabilitation Studies Handbook*. Cambridge: Cambridge University Press.

McMillan, T. M. and Sparkes, C. (1999). Goal planning and neurorehabilitation: the Wolfson Neurorehabilitation Centre approach. *Neuropsychological Rehabilitation*, *9*(3/4), 241–251.

Melville, L. L., Baltic, T. A., Bettcher, T. W. and Nelson, D. L. (2002). Patients' perspectives on the self-identified goals assessment. *American Journal of Occupational Therapy*, *56*(6), 650–659.

Monaghan, J., Channell, K., McDowell, D. and Sharma, A. (2005). Improving patient and carer communication, multidisciplinary team working and goal-setting in stroke rehabilitation. *Clinical Rehabilitation*, *19*(2), 194–199.

Nair, K. P. S. (2003). Life goals: the concept and its relevance to rehabilitation. *Clinical Rehabilitation*, *17*, 192–202.

Nair, K. P. S. and Wade, D. T. (2003). Life goals of people with disabilities due to neurological disorders. *Clinical Rehabilitation*, *17*(5), 521–527.

Pendleton, H. M. and Schultz-Krohn, W. (2005). *Pedretti's Occupational Therapy Practice Skills for Physical Dysfunction (6th edn)*. St Louis, MO: Mosby Elsevier.

Petrie, K. J., Cameron, L. D., Ellis, C. J., Buick, D. and Weinman J. (2002). Changing illness perceptions following myocardial infarction: an early intervention randomized controlled trial. *Psychosomatic Medicine*, *64*, 580–586.

Phipps, S. and Richardson, P. (2007). Occupational therapy outcomes for clients with traumatic brain injury and stroke using the Canadian Occupational Performance Measure. *American Journal of Occupational Therapy*, *61*(3), 328–334.

Playford, E. D., Dawson, L., Limbert, V., Smith, M., Ward, C. D. and Wells, R. (2000). Goal-setting in rehabilitation: report of a workshop to explore professionals' perceptions of goal-setting. *Clinical Rehabilitation*, *14*(5), 491–496.

Powell, J., Heslin, J. and Greenwood, R. (2002). Community based rehabilitation after severe traumatic brain injury: a randomised controlled trial. *Journal of Neurology, Neurosurgery and Psychiatry*, *72*(2), 193–202.

Randall, K. E. and McEwen, I. R. (2000). Writing patient-centered functional goals. *Physical Therapy*, *80*(12), 1197–1203.

Rauch, A., Cieza, A. and Stucki, G. (2008). How to apply the International Classification of Functioning, Disability and Health (ICF) for rehabilitation management in clinical practice. *European Journal of Physical and Rehabilitation Medicine*, *44*(3), 329–342.

Rubin, R. S. (2002). Will the real SMART goals please stand up? *The Industrial-Organisational Psychologist*, *39*(4), 26–27. http://siop.org/tip/backissues/TIPApr02//03rubin.aspx (accessed 15 February 2011).

Salter, K., Helling, C., Foley, N. and Teasell, R. (2008). The experience of living with stroke: a qualitative meta-synthesis. *Journal of Rehabilitation Medicine*, *40*, 595–602.

Schut, H. A. and Stam, H. J. (1994). Goals in rehabilitation teamwork. *Disability and Rehabilitation*, *16*(4), 223–226.

Scofield, M. E., Pape, D. A., McCracken, N. and Maki, D. R. (1980). An ecological model of promoting acceptance of disability. *Journal of Applied Rehabilitation Counseling*, *11*, 183–187.

Scott, I. A. (2010). Preventing the rebound: improving care transistion in hospital discharge process. *Australian Health Review*, *34*, 445–451.

Sigelman, C. K., Vengroff, L. P. and Spanhell, C. L. (1979). Disability and the concept of life functions. *Rehabilitation Counseling Bulletin*, *23*, 103–113.

Sullivan, M. J., Adams, H., Rhodenizer, T. and Stanish, W. D. (2006). A psychosocial risk factor–targeted intervention for the prevention of chronic pain and disability following whiplash injury. *Physical Therapy*, *86*(1), 8–18.

Tripp, S. (1999). Providing psychological support. In: M. Smith (Editor). *Rehabilitation in Adult Nursing Practice*. Edinburgh: Churchill Livingstone, pp. 105–112.

Trombly, C. A. and Wu, C.Y. (1999). Effect of rehabilitation tasks on organization of movement after stroke. *American Journal of Occupational Therapy*, *53*(4), 333–344.

Trombly, C. A., Radomski, M. V., Trexel, C. and Burnet-Smith, S. E. (2002). Occupational therapy and achievement of self-identified goals by adults with acquired brain injury: phase II. *American Journal of Occupational Therapy*, *56*(5), 489–498.

Turner-Stokes, L. (2009). Goal attainment scaling (GAS) in rehabilitation: a practical guide. *Clinical Rehabilitation*, *23*, 362–370.

Turner-Stokes, L. and Williams, H. (2010). Goal attainment scaling: a direct comparison of alternative rating methods. *Clinical Rehabilitation*, *24*, 66–73.

Turner, B. J., Fleming, J.M., Ownsworth, T. L. and Cornwell, P. L. (2008). The transistion from hospital to home for individuals with acquired brain injury: a literature review and research recommendations. *Disability and Rehabilitation*, *30*(16), 1153–1176.

Wade, D. T. (1998). Evidence relating to goal planning in rehabilitation. *Clinical Rehabilitation*, *12*(4), 273–275.

Wade, D. T. (1999a). Goal planning in stroke rehabilitation: why? *Topics in Stroke Rehabilitation*, *6*(2), 1–7.

Wade, D. T. (1999b). Goal planning in stroke rehabilitation: how? *Topics in Stroke Rehabilitation*, *6*(2), 16–36.

Wade, D. T. (2005). Describing rehabilitation interventions. *Clinical Rehabilitation*, *19*, 811–818.

Wade, D. T. (2009). Goal setting in rehabilitation: an overview of what, why and how. *Clinical Rehabilitation*, *23*, 291–295.

Wade, D. T., Smeets, R. J. E. M. and Verbunt, J. A. (2010). Research in rehabilitation medicine: methodological challenges. *Journal of Clinical Epidemiology*, *63*, 699–704.

Whiteneck, G., Dijkers, M., Gassaway, J. and Lammertse, D. P. (2009). The SCI Rehab Project: classification and quantification of spinal cord injury rehabilitation treatments. *Journal of Spinal Cord Medicine*, *32*(3), 249–250.

Wilson, B. A. (2008). Neuropsychological rehabilitation. *Annual Review of Clinical Psychology*, *4*, 141–162.

World Health Organization. (2001). *International Classification of Functioning, Disability and Health: ICF*. Geneva: WHO.

Wressle, E., Eeg-Olofsson, A. M., Marcusson, A. M. and Henriksson, C. (2002). Improved client participation in the rehabilitation process using a client-centred goal formulation structure. *Journal of Rehabilitation Medicine*, *34*(1), 5–11.

Ylvisaker, M. and Feeney, T. (2000). Reconstruction of identity after traumatic brain injury. *Brain Impairment*, *1*, 12–28.

Ylvisaker, M. and Feeney, T. (2002). Executive functions, self-regulation, and learned optimism in paediatric rehabilitation: a review and implications for intervention. *Pediatric Rehabilitation*, *5*(2), 51–70.

Ylvisaker, M., McPherson, K., Kayes, N. and Pellett, E. (2008). Metaphoric identity mapping: facilitating goal setting and engagement in rehabilitation after traumatic brain injury. *Neuropsychological Rehabilitation*, *18*(5–6), 713–741.

Chapter 5

Outcome measurement in rehabilitation

Richard J. Siegert[1] and Jo Adams[2]

[1] *Professor of Psychology and Rehabilitation, School of Rehabilitation and Occupation Studies and School of Public Health and Psychosocial Studies, AUT University, Auckland, New Zealand;* [2] *Senior Lecturer and Professional Lead for Occupational Therapy, Faculty of Health Sciences, University of Southampton, United Kingdom*

5.1   Introduction

How often have you been asked recently to participate in a research study, a political poll or a customer satisfaction survey? We live in an age that is obsessed with information, counting and measurement. Much of this preoccupation with numbers and facts is due to the invention of the modern, high-speed computer, which makes collecting and analysing information so easy. However, at times it can feel as if we are being assailed by facts and figures, rather than helped by them. We feel swamped with information and ideas but short of time to assimilate all this information and reflect upon its implications. In the clinical environment busy health professionals can sometimes feel besieged by institutional requirements to collect data on their daily activities. At the same time there is constant pressure on health professionals to keep up to date with the growing amount of new information in their field and the implications of all this new knowledge for everyday patient care.

This chapter is about measurement in rehabilitation and how we measure the results or *outcomes* of the process of rehabilitation. It is also about how we decide which measure or measures are the best to use for our specific purpose and targeted interventions. In particular we consider the best ways to measure the outcomes of interprofessional rehabilitation while keeping the individual client's or patient's perspective as the central focus.

An outcome in rehabilitation has been defined as 'a characteristic or construct that is expected to change owing to the strategy, intervention, or program' (Finch et al., 2002, p. 11). Another definition states that: 'Outcome refers to the expected or looked for change in some measure or state. In other words, a patient will enter a rehabilitation

Interprofessional Rehabilitation: A Person-Centred Approach, First Edition.
Edited by Sarah G. Dean, Richard J. Siegert and William J. Taylor.
© 2012 John Wiley & Sons, Ltd. Published 2012 by John Wiley & Sons, Ltd.

program in one state and may change as a result of the intervention. The new state constitutes this outcome' (Wade, 2003, p. 27).

Finch et al. (2002) suggest that three measurement paradigms with particular relevance to evaluating rehabilitation outcomes are (1) the World Health Organization's (WHO) International Classification of Functioning, Disability and Health (ICF), (2) health-related quality of life (HRQoL), and (3) cost. Finch and colleagues note that outcomes can be targeted at the level of the organ, the person or the group, and they argue that the ideal outcome to measure is one that is most affected by our strategy, intervention or programme and minimally affected by other influences. Outcomes need to be measured in some way by clinicians and this just means that a set measurement tool (for example a standardized questionnaire, functional test or goniometer) is used to quantify these observations (Barnes and Ward, 2000).

This chapter will attempt to address a number of specific, important and complex questions about rehabilitation outcome measures. Specifically it will attempt to address the following questions.

• Why do we use outcome measures?
• What are the important outcomes to measure?
• Who decides *what* to measure?
• What makes a 'good' measure?
• How can we best apply outcome measures in clinical practice?
• How should outcome measurement influence practice and service delivery?

Why do we use outcome measures in rehabilitation?

A recent survey of New Zealand physiotherapists treating patients with low back pain, found that the majority of the therapists did not routinely or systematically use standardized outcome measures in their day-to-day clinical practice, preferring instead to rely upon their individual clinical judgement and the patient's verbal report (Copeland et al., 2008). Interestingly, this finding is not unique with similar results reported in studies from Scotland, Canada and the USA (Chesson et al., 1996; Huijbregts et al., 2002; Jette et al., 2009). Given such findings, one might reasonably ask why already busy rehabilitation clinicians would want to add to their workload by making data collection on outcome measures a routine part of their clinical practice? In fact there are important ethical, clinical, financial and scientific reasons why outcome measures are useful and important for routine practice in rehabilitation settings. But underpinning all these reasons is the prevailing belief that the patient's voice must be heard and should feature in any consideration of health outcomes. This makes sense, as rehabilitation professionals we treat the individual and not simply the condition.

Ultimately how the patient feels they are progressing or coping is paramount. In both the UK and the USA it has been generally accepted that it is important to obtain the patient's view on therapy outcome and governments have endorsed recommendations to increase the use of patient reported outcome measures in documenting the effectiveness of health services (Marshall et al., 2005; US Department of Health and

Table 5.1   Taxonomy of applications of patient-reported outcome (PRO) in clinical practice. (From Greenhalgh, 2009. Reproduced with kind permission from Springer Science + Business Media.)

		Level of aggregation of PRO data	
		Individual	**Group**
Used at the clinician–patient interface	**Yes**	Screening Monitoring Promoting patient-centred care	Decision aids
	No	Facilitating communication within multidisciplinary teams	Population monitoring and assessing quality of care

Human Services Food and Drug Administration, 2009). Increasingly you will see and hear the term 'patient-reported outcome measures' (PROMs) to refer to tools designed to collect information on what patients think about their therapy progress, their health status and the quality of service delivery. Greenhalgh (2009) has recently proposed a taxonomy or system for classifying the different applications PROM data can be used for (see Table 5.1, Greenhalgh, 2009). In this taxonomy PROMs are classified according to two dimensions. The first dimension is based upon whether or not a person's scores on the measure are used at the level of the individual patient–clinician interaction. The second dimension is concerned with whether patient scores on the measure are considered as individual or grouped data.

Greenhalgh observes that individual PROM data can be used in the clinician–patient interaction for (1) screening, (2) monitoring, and (3) promoting patient-centred care. Screening involves using a standardized PROM, with all patients in a service, as a diagnostic aid for detecting problems in individuals that are frequently not diagnosed. For example, depression is common in neurological rehabilitation and the Beck Depression Inventory (BDI) is a popular screening tool (Siegert et al., 2009, 2010). If a patient scores above a certain cut-off point on the BDI there is a high probability of a mood disorder and further investigation is warranted. Monitoring refers to the ongoing observation and measurement of specific aspects of a patient's condition or life circumstances to see if things are improving, deteriorating or remain about the same. For example, the Palliative care Outcome Scale (POS) is a brief, 10-item questionnaire that monitors important aspects of a patient's comfort, clinical care and psychological/spiritual well-being in palliative care settings (Hearn & Higginson, 1999; Siegert et al., 2010).

Promoting patient-centred care means that a measure is used to foster patient self-management of their health and to encourage patients to become active partners in the long-term management of their health. This is particularly important in rehabilitation where people must be actively engaged in the process for it to be at all effective. PROMs can assist this process by helping to ensure that patients participate in determining the important goals for their own treatment. For example, the WHOQOL-BREF is a self-report measure that asks people about physical, psychological, social and environmental dimensions of their overall quality of life (QoL). It can be used to monitor changes in QoL in the management of chronic health conditions such as rheumatoid arthritis (Taylor et al., 2004).

Greenhalgh's (2009) taxonomy also includes those situations in which individual PROM data is used without a patient–clinician interaction occurring. An example is when individual PROM scores are used to facilitate communication about patients within a multidisciplinary team. For example, an inpatient team on a specialized neurorehabilitation ward might use a measure such as the Functional Independence Measure + Functional Assessment Measure – UK version (UK FIM+FAM) at fortnightly team meetings to consider the progress of each patient (Turner-Stokes et al., 1999). The FIM+FAM serves as both a focus for discussion and a shared framework for all disciplines to co-ordinate their diverse skills and knowledge in assisting each individual patient toward greater independence. It has two subscales that measure physical and cognitive disability/independence and can highlight the specific targets for rehabilitation necessary to achieve greater independence before discharge from an inpatient service. It can also serve to remind the team when an individual patient is not making the progress expected and so indicate when some concerted clinical problem solving is required.

Two other uses for PROMs data that emerged from this typology involved the use of grouped, rather than individual, data. Grouped data refers to when patients are studied as part of an audit, research project or service evaluation and offers generalized indications about how groups of individuals respond to a certain intervention. Such information can help clinicians review the effectiveness of interventions and help guide decisions about service planning – such as deciding which interventions are most effective for which patients. This is particularly relevant when results from randomized controlled trials are used to help individual patients and their clinicians make decisions concerning their own treatment or clinical management. For example, patients considering undergoing cancer treatments that have unpleasant side-effects can be informed about patient data on QoL from trials of these treatments.

The second use of grouped PROM data is for 'evaluating the effectiveness of routine care and assessing the quality of care' (Greenhalgh, 2009, p. 118). For example the Services Obstacles Scale (SOS) is a brief (six item) questionnaire that was developed to provide information on the barriers to rehabilitation services in the community that people with a traumatic brain injury have experienced (Kolakowsky-Hayner et al., 2000; Marwitz and Kreutzer, 1996).

Implicit in the above discussion of PROMs is the notion that using them will necessarily improve the quality of the service and care provided. In other words it is assumed that the collection of PROM data will somehow change clinician behaviour and spur people into action to improve the delivery of care. But is there any evidence to support this? The best current evidence available does not allow a simple yes or no answer to this question. Two recent reviews observed that there was good evidence that feedback from PROMs often has positive effects such as improving diagnosis (especially in mental health settings) and improving clinician–patient communication – but it remains to be established whether regular use of PROMs has a substantial impact on the health of most patients (Skinner and Turner-Stokes, 2006; Valderas et al., 2008; Greenhalgh, 2009).

What are the important outcomes to measure?

As society progresses, definitions of health and well-being also evolve – reflecting current knowledge and expectations as well as changing political, economic and social influences. Outcome measures have developed from being rather narrow, biomedical indicators of outcome, such as statistics on death, disease and disability, to include much broader instruments that attempt to capture the individual's personal and subjective experience of disability, health and well-being. There has been a continuing evolution of healthcare definitions and the language used to capture ability and function. Today the focus on recording outcomes is much more on people's abilities and their role in society rather than just on their symptoms and limitations.

In deciding what are the important outcomes to measure in rehabilitation there are two key issues that we need to consider from the outset. The first issue is precisely *which level of functioning* is most appropriate or relevant to assess in measuring outcome. This is important because it makes sense to measure outcomes at the level at which our therapy or intervention is targeted. In rehabilitation we are fortunate to have a sophisticated conceptual framework developed by the WHO that enables us to categorize and compartmentalize most elements of a person's daily function – the ICF (WHO, 2001). The second issue here concerns who decides *what the important outcomes to measure are* in the first place? Is it the patient, the family, the clinician, the service manager, the funder or government? This question of 'important to whom?' is arguably the single most important issue in outcome measurement. However, to answer this important question, it is helpful to first understand where the ICF fits in to outcome measurement and how outcome measures relate to the ICF model.

ICF level of functioning and outcome measurement

Derick Wade has argued persuasively that the WHO model of health, disability and functioning provides an excellent conceptual framework for clinicians to match up their interventions with appropriate outcome measures (Wade, 1991). The WHO model has been developed and refined further since Wade's influential text on measurement in neurological rehabilitation was first published and the current version is presented earlier (see Chapter 2, Figure 2.1). The important point about the ICF in relation to outcome measures is that it requires a clinician to specify at which level (body functions and structures, activities, participation, environmental and personal factors) they intend to intervene and to measure their effectiveness at that level. So if we intervene at the level of body structures and functions, such as muscle strengthening in physiotherapy, then clearly we need an outcome measure that operates at this level. In contrast, if we use social skills training to increase vocational involvement in people recovering from severe traumatic brain injury (TBI), then we need to measure outcome at the participation level.

But rehabilitation is a complex intervention and typically involves multiple professionals working with a patient and their family/carers over several months and sometimes years. Moreover an intervention can be highly specific, such as a single session of occupational therapy focused on dressing oneself, or it can be comprehensive, such as a community-based programme supporting the families of people with a TBI. Wade suggests that it is nevertheless important to be specific and 'refer to the outcome of a specified intervention measured in a specific way, reflecting the interests of specific groups/stakeholders...' (Wade, 2003, p. 27).

In other words before we dare to inflict a new outcome measure on our clients, patients or colleagues we should always be able to specify the following features of our outcome measurement plan:

- the intervention that we are interested in evaluating;
- the level of function, in ICF terms, where this intervention is believed to have an impact;
- the proposed outcome measure that captures change at this level of function;
- and who identified this outcome as the important one?

In practice this will often demand that we measure outcomes at more than one ICF level or domain. A good example of this comes from the progress that has been made in upper limb surgery for tetraplegia since the early 1980s. There is substantial evidence from case series that forearm tendon transfer surgery can produce improved fine arm–hand functioning in people with tetraplegia and that these gains are maintained over time (Rothwell et al., 2003). However, most of the outcome research on this surgery has focused exclusively on direct improvements in hand function such as hook grip and pinch grip values. These are measurements at the level of body structures and functions and research has focused on this level because it is here that hand surgeons have been able to directly evaluate their success. However, recent approaches to evaluating the success of this type of hand surgery have focused more on how the surgery has affected the person at the participation level (Sinnott et al., 2009). For example, the following quote is from a person who had the surgery a few years ago: 'I think the surgery has helped my level of confidence. For example when I go out in public I can be sure of managing a cup of coffee and eating with a fork. These things help with self-esteem. It also means I can do more for myself and other people...' (Sinnott et al., 2004, p. 398).

This kind of outcome information is important for people who might be weighing up whether or not to have the surgery but also for administrators who might be considering how many operations to fund each year. The point here is that we often need to evaluate outcomes at different levels and the ICF provides a useful conceptual framework for doing this. This example also illustrates the point that different outcomes matter more or less for different stakeholders. Similarly, there are many outcome measures that could be considered for the following case study and possible outcome measure options using the WHO model of health, disability and functioning framework are considered here.

Case study: part 1

A 52-year-old shop worker, Jackie, has been diagnosed with sero-positive rheumatoid arthritis following a 15-month history of pain, swelling and early morning stiffness of varying severity affecting her knees, wrists, small finger joints and metatarsals. She is now struggling to sleep and finding that she is tired and fatigued throughout the day. Her functional ability at home and at work is limited by her pain and stiffness in her upper limbs. Jackie is using her non-steroidal anti-inflammatory drugs and pain medications daily as prescribed to control her pain but has not sought any other intervention for pain relief.

The disease activity of the underlying inflammatory disease process (body function) would be appropriate to initially screen and monitor. A well-validated, well-used international example of this could be the 28 Joint Disease Activity Score (Prevoo, 1995). This is a simple measure of the tenderness and swelling of 28 joints computed with erythrocyte sedimentation rates (full details of which can be found at http://www.das-score.nl/). If we want to ensure that the individual is included in contributing to this level of body function assessment a simple 100 mm anchored visual analogue scale (VAS) of specific joint pain and swelling ranging from 0 = no pain/swelling to 100 mm = extreme pain or swelling could also be utilized. For screening of body structures to obtain baseline information for suitability of intervention such as orthotics or an exercise prescription a site-specific outcome measure could be used. An example of a structural joint scale, examining the wrist and hand collecting ratio data, is the Total Active Motion Scale (Spiegel et al., 1987). This records the total active range of the joint in question. A clinician-assessed standardized functional assessment could complement this. The Grip Ability Test (Dellhag and Bjelle, 1995) is one such outcome. We will return to this case later in this Chapter to complete the picture of possible options for outcome measurements for Jackie.

QoL in rehabilitation

One important concept in modern health sciences that does not feature prominently in the ICF is the construct of QoL (Fayers and Machin, 2007; Leplege and Hunt, 1997). The ICF is largely concerned with *function* or what a person can do whereas QoL is more concerned with overall how happy or satisfied a person feels about their life at this point in time. The concept of function is relatively objective – we can observe if a person can walk, talk, get dressed, drive a car or earn a living. In contrast the notion of QoL is entirely subjective – only the individual can say how happy they are with their current lot in life. QoL is notoriously difficult to define or rather it is difficult to find a definition that everyone can agree on. Calman asserted that QoL must take into account numerous aspects of a person's life and that only the individual can report on their own QoL. Calman argued for a model in which QoL is conceptualized as the difference between a person's hopes and expectations and their present lived experience (Calman, 1984). The WHO defines QoL as 'individuals' perception of their position in life in the context of the culture and value systems in which they live and in relation to their goals, expectations, standards and concerns' (Division of Mental Health and Prevention of Substance Abuse, 1997, p. 1). The WHO definition is the basis of the WHOQOL measure and posits six important dimensions or domains of QoL – physical health, psychological, level of independence, social relationships, environment and spirituality/religion/personal beliefs. However, because it is so difficult to adequately define QoL most workers in the field prefer to use the more limited term Health Related Quality of Life (HRQOL) (Fayers and Machin, 2007). HRQoL measures can be divided into generic and disease-specific HRQoL measures. One example of a generic HRQoL measure is the Short Form-36 (SF-36) that has been used to gauge QoL in a broad range of health conditions as well as in healthy people (Quality Metric, n.d.). In contrast the QOLIE-89 was specifically developed to measure QoL in people with epilepsy (Devinsky et al., 1995). The strength of a disease-specific instrument is that the items are developed with input from people with the condition concerned, resulting in a set of items with direct relevance to people with that condition. The strength of more generic instruments is that they can be used to compare QoL across people with different conditions.

Who decides which outcomes are the important ones?

We already know that patients' and health professionals' perspectives of disease and functional ability often differ (Nothnagl et al., 2005; Salaffi et al., 2005) so relying solely on clinician-rated measures gives only a limited view of rehabilitation outcome. If we accept that health is a subjective concept, dependent upon physical, cognitive and emotional factors, and affected by social, economic and geographic influences, then it is clear how important it is to obtain a patient's perspective on their own state of health and progress in rehabilitation.

A recent qualitative study that looked at the views of patients towards two widely used back pain outcome measures concluded that both of these measures were inadequate from a patient perspective. The measures were criticized for not fully capturing the personal experiences of living and working with back pain and for not addressing all of the most relevant changes that can occur with this condition (Hush et al., 2010). The study also criticized these measures in relation to the time frame for assessment and the functional domains covered. It would be premature and unwise to discard two well-established measures on the basis of a single study that included only 36 participants from one country, but the study does illustrate some important trends in rehabilitation outcomes.

However, to get a better picture and understanding of the impact of a condition we need to consider using PROMS and, using the example of our earlier case about Jackie, there would be a number available to us. These could be either generic or site and/or disease specific.

Case study: part 2

For Jackie it may be appropriate to use a generic disease-specific measure such as the Arthritis Impact Measurement Scale (AIMS, Meenan, 1982) or the Health Assessment Questionnaire (HAQ, Fries et al., 1980). These would help gain insight into baseline levels of functional (dis)ability. Both of these measures are internationally used and have good levels of reliability and validity in arthritis populations. If we were concerned to assess general functional ability in a tailored manner, so that we are able to discern more specifically which daily tasks are particularly troublesome for Jackie then it may be that the Personal Impact Health Assessment Questionnaire (PI-HAQ, Hewlett et al., 2002) could be another useful option.

When deciding which outcome measures to use it would be useful to consider how a tool was developed and who was included in the construction and testing of the tool. The development of an outcome measure should ideally include groups of patients and clinical specialists to decide which are the most relevant and pertinent questions to ask and how the outcome should be framed. Patients need to be asked what matters most to them and what issues are the most important that need to be addressed in a measure. A sound outcome measure will have been developed using committees of experts in the field that include patients (and or family/carers), clinicians and academics. Ensuring that patients are consulted at all stages in the development and refinement of outcome measures is essential.

It may also be necessary for outcome measures to be updated at regular intervals so that items or questions do not become out of date and to ensure that they accurately reflect contemporary lifestyles and values. One example of this is the work conducted by Stamm and colleagues exploring the usefulness of standardized questionnaires used to assess people with hand-based osteoarthritis (Stamm et al., 2009). This team explored whether the concepts important to patients with hand osteoarthritis (OA) were covered by the most commonly used outcome measures. Only a third of the concepts identified by patients with hand OA as important were covered by those standardized questionnaires in common use. None of these questionnaires considered how having hand OA had psychological consequences, the different qualities of pain, aesthetic changes or impact on leisure activities – all of which were identified as important by this patient group. In addition the outcome measures were seen to be out-dated by the patients. For example, some important activities such as using a mobile phone and caring for grandchildren, were not represented in these outcome measures, which had been developed several years ago.

What makes a good outcome measure?

Once we have decided *what* the important things to measure are then we need to decide *how* we intend to measure them. In practice this usually means deciding which tool, scale or measure is the best instrument available for measuring those outcomes we have decided are most important. Unfortunately, choosing just which outcome measure to use in any clinical context is not a simple matter, due in part to the growing number of these measures now available. For example, a systematic review of measures of anxiety and depression suitable for use with people with a spinal cord injury compared 12 different instruments reported in the literature (Sakakibara et al., 2009). Another systematic review that considered measures of walking and mobility in neurological conditions found 17 separate measures (Tyson, 2009). So how does a busy clinician select the best outcome measure from 12 or 17 separate measures? This issue involves the technical aspects of measurement development known as *psychometrics* (Nunnally and Bernstein, 1994). Psychometrics is a field that first developed in education and psychology in the late 19th and throughout the 20th Century (Anastasi and Urbina, 1997). In both of these fields the measurement of individual differences were important concerns and there now exists a sophisticated range of statistical techniques for developing and evaluating robust measurement tools. In the next section we will introduce some of the major concepts that underpin the field known as psychometrics. However, this is a large and rather technical topic, well beyond the scope of the present text and the interested reader is referred to a number of good texts on psychometrics at the end of this chapter.

5.2   Psychometrics – a primer

Some of the key terms that are necessary to understand when evaluating any outcome measure are *utility, reliability, validity* and *responsiveness*. However, the first term that we need to consider here is *measurement*.

Measurement

At its simplest measurement can be described as a process for assigning attributes to objects (Nunnally and Bernstein, 1994). For example height, weight and body temperature are all attributes that can be assigned to people. Similarly volume, mass and temperature are attributes that can be assigned to characterize people, objects, living organisms and planets. Moreover, when we assign a height or weight to an individual we assume that there is a simple and consistent relationship between their height or weight and the scale used to measure the attribute. In other words we expect somebody who is measured at 72 cm to be the same height as every other 72 cm tall person on the planet – even though they might differ in gender, weight, ethnicity, eye colour or any other measureable attribute. What is more we expect the centimetre intervals on our ruler or measuring tape to all be exactly the same length. But is this also the case when we try to measure such elusive concepts as anxiety, QoL, participation, community integration and spiritual well-being?

In the jargon of statisticians such constructs are known as *latent variables* – a term that describes variables that cannot be directly observed and hence are inferred or measured indirectly. For example, we cannot touch, see or count 'depression', so to measure depression in a person, we ask a series of questions about different aspects of the construct and we infer the presence or absence of depression based upon the answers to those questions. To quantify the latent variable we assign a number to the answers to those questions and add all the resulting numbers together to give a total score indicative of how depressed the person is. Adding or summing the numerical values of the responses to all the items or questions on a measure implies that the measure is a *scale*. However, a scale of anxiety or QoL is very different from a ruler or bathroom scales. What does it really mean to say that a person's self-reported QoL has improved from 18 to 24 on a scale that ranges from 0 to 30? Is this the same improvement as another patient whose score rose from 10 to 16? Indeed ask yourself what it would mean if a patient actually reported zero or 30 on the same scale? The need to measure latent variables is in part why the field of psychometrics developed rapidly in the 20th century and continues to be a rapidly evolving field today. Those readers interested in a critical and sceptical approach to the scientific basis of psychometrics should acquaint themselves with the writings of psychologist Joel Michell (1990, 2000).

Utility

This refers to the practical (and non-statistical) characteristics of a measurement tool – such as how much time it takes to complete and whether it has to be paid for or if it is available free. Utility is arguably the most important consideration of all since a tool that has poor utility will not be widely used regardless of how good its statistical properties are. Service managers will not be interested in outcome measures that are expensive and clinicians and patients do not have time for lengthy or complicated measures. If the tool is completed by or with patients then it is essential to consider the extent of 'patient burden' involved in data collection. In practice this means that a PROM should be simple and clear, in both language and format, and it should be as brief as possible. A recent review of literacy levels required to complete some PROMs suggest that many require university-level reading ability for patients to fully understand them (Adams et al., 2009). If patients are unable to understand the questions we ask then the quality of their responses is likely to be compromised. In reviewing the utility of a measurement tool try to find PROMs that are brief to complete, use simple sentences, have plenty of space between the questions and use very few polysyllabic words.

From the perspective of the health professional it must also be easy to score and interpret and provide information on important variables. There are numerous examples where longer, comprehensive tools have been successfully shortened. In upper limb rehabilitation the Disability of the Arm Shoulder and Hand (DASH) Questionnaire (Hudak et al., 1996) is a well-respected tool that has been popular across many orthopaedic and vocational rehabilitation programmes. More recently, the Quick DASH (Beaton et al., 2005) has been developed. This is a quicker, short version with better utility for the patient and clinician. It is also just as robust from a measurement point of view as the longer version (Whalley and Adams, 2009) and can serve as an excellent resource for busy clinicians.

In rehabilitation settings it is particularly important to consider the influence of any sensory or cognitive impairments that might prevent a patient from filling out a measure or providing accurate information. For example, in the Regional Rehabilitation Unit (RRU) at Northwick Park Hospital the BDI is used to screen for depression in neurorehabilitation patients, many of whom have sensory/cognitive/communication impairments (Siegert et al., 2009, 2010). Under normal circumstances a person can complete this 21-item pencil and paper questionnaire in a few minutes. At Northwick Park RRU a large print version of the BDI-II is used for patients with such impairments and items are presented to individual patients one at a time and read aloud by the psychologist. The response options are presented with each item and also read out loud. The administration is done as slowly as required according to the patient's condition and items/response options are repeated as often as is necessary. On some occasions a speech and language therapist will assist the clinical psychologist administering the BDI-II.

Reliability

This refers to how accurate or precise the scores we get from an outcome measure are. In the same way that we rely upon our bathroom scales or our car's speedometer to give us accurate readings – we also need to be sure that our outcome scores can be relied upon. However, there are different approaches to reliability. One form of reliability is called *internal consistency* and this is concerned with the extent to which all the items or questions in a single measure are correlated with each other. This type of reliability is measured by a statistic known as the coefficient alpha or Cronbach's alpha (Streiner, 2003). This statistic, represented by the Greek symbol α, can range from 0 to 1 and satisfactory internal consistency is usually taken as falling between 0.70 and 0.95 (Streiner, 2003). An outcome measure with a large α is regarded as a relatively homogeneous measure or one where all the items are tapping into aspects of the same construct. However, some measurement tools are not homogeneous and have two or more subscales within them. For example, the Hospital Anxiety and Depression Scale (HADS) has two subscales as its names suggests, one for anxiety and one for depression (Zigmond and Snaith, 1983). When a measure has two or more subscales then we are more interested in the internal consistency of the individual subscales so the test authors should report Cronbach's α for each subscale as well as for the entire scale. Internal consistency or Cronbach's α is calculated using the test scores of a large number of people who each completed the outcome measure on a single occasion.

There is another very important class of reliability that is concerned with how consistent scores on a measure are for the same person across time or across different people using the same rating scale.[1] These two different aspects of reliability are referred to as *test–retest* and *inter-rater* reliability. Test–retest reliability is concerned with the notion that a person's total score on a measure should not change dramatically in a short space of time (unless of course their clinical condition changes dramatically). This form of reliability is measured simply by administering the same measure on two occasions (often about 3–7 days apart) to a group of people and calculating the correlation between test scores at time 1 and time 2. Test–retest reliability is usually considered good for clinical purposes if the correlation between the total scores on the two occasions is ≥ 0.80.

Inter-rater reliability concerns those measures where one person rates or completes a measure for another person. For example, the FIM is widely used in rehabilitation

---

[1] Just to complicate things there is another type of reliability known as *parallel forms*. This is when two or more equivalent forms of the same measure exist and the correlation between these parallel forms can be calculated. Parallel forms are quite common in achievement tests (e.g. mathematics, science) but less common in rehabilitation. One setting where parallel tests are used is in clinical neuropsychology to examine things like vocabulary, verbal memory, arithmetic and general knowledge. This is to prevent 'practice effects' where people improve simply through previous exposure to the test questions.

to measure how independent patients are in their activities of daily living and is typically completed by a health professional. Inter-rater reliability is concerned with how closely two different health professionals will rate the same patient. It is usually calculated by getting two or more trained raters to independently rate the same group of individual patients and then calculating the level of agreement using an intra-class correlation coefficient (ICC, Streiner and Norman, 2008). Measures of reliability offer no indication of the validity of the measure however, and cannot give any information about just what is being measured.

Validity

The validity of an outcome measure is the extent to which that measure actually measures what it is supposed to measure. For example, the validity of a measure of participation (in ICF terms) is the extent to which we can be confident that this measure actually captures in numerical form most of the important elements of participation. Streiner and Norman note that historically validity has been conceptualized in terms of the 'three Cs'- *content* validity, *criterion* validity and *construct* validity (Streiner and Norman, 2008).

Content validity

A measure that has good content validity is one that systematically covers all the important, diverse aspects of the construct we are trying to measure. In the past when you have sat an examination you will have been concerned with the content validity of that exam. In other words the exam should (1) only contain questions about subject matter that featured in the course you just took, (2) it should systematically cover most of the important topics taught, and (3) it must not examine you on topics that were not in the course. To take a clinical example, a questionnaire designed to assess anxiety should ask questions about all the important symptom dimensions that characterize anxiety. These would include physical symptoms (e.g. *Does your heart race or pound for no reason?*), cognitive symptoms (e.g. *Do you spend time worrying about things?*) and behavioural symptoms (e.g. *Do you avoid social gatherings?*).

Criterion validity

This refers to the extent to which a measure relates strongly to other ways of measuring the same or closely related constructs. Ideally there is a 'gold standard' for measuring the construct we wish to measure and this can be compared or correlated with our measure. For example, the development of new measures of anxiety and depression frequently involves comparing scores on these measures with the results of a psychiatric interview, which is considered the gold standard. However, often there is no gold standard for a concept or construct and so test developers make do by comparing their new measure with a range of other existing measures. These existing measures may have been used with good effect in other specialities, with different patient groups or with different communities but just not applied in the specific area of interest. Generally, in these situations the new measure has some added advantage over the existing ones, such as being briefer or more comprehensive; otherwise we might question the need for another measure of the same construct. Authorities on psychometrics often divide criterion validity in to two types – *concurrent* and *predictive validity* (Bowling, 2005; Streiner and Norman, 2008). Concurrent validity means correlating a questionnaire or rating scale with other such measures at one point in time i.e. a cross-sectional study. For example, Siegert and colleagues developed a brief social support questionnaire and validated it by correlating it with two other existing measures of social support that both focused on somewhat different aspects of this multidimensional construct (Siegert et al., 1987). Predictive validity, as its name suggests, is concerned with how well scores on a scale can predict some future event such as length of stay in an in-patient rehabilitation unit or returning to work. For example, the Glasgow Coma Scale (GCS) is a popular rating scale that is widely used to assess the level of consciousness in people after a head injury or other trauma (Teasdale and Jennett, 1974). The GCS has three domains – eye-opening, verbal and motor responses – and patients are given a score for each resulting in a total score that can range from 3 to 15. No doubt the popularity of the GCS is due in large part to its utility. It takes only a few minutes to complete, requires minimal training and can easily be administered at the bedside by a nurse or roadside by paramedics. This makes it a practical and popular index of clinical severity in acute trauma settings all over the world. But the other reason for its sustained popularity over several decades now is its predictive value. There is substantial evidence that the GCS is a useful predictor of variables such as hospital mortality, duration of coma and post-traumatic amnesia (PTA) and long-term outcomes after discharge (Zuercher et al., 2009). In other words the GCS has well-established predictive validity.

Construct validity

Construct validity is concerned with the theory behind a measure and with how well the measure reflects that theory. It is also about how scores on the measure relate to other relevant variables and the extent to which these relationships support or refute the theory behind the measure. Much of the time in rehabilitation we are concerned with measuring outcomes in terms of complex concepts such as QoL, participation, community integration, executive functioning and dignity. These are abstract or theoretical constructs that we attempt to measure using a questionnaire or rating scale that has multiple items that are designed to tap all the diverse aspects of the underlying construct. In psychometric jargon the construct that is reflected in the items of a questionnaire is often called a *factor* or a *latent variable*.

A statistical technique known as factor analysis is often used as one line of evidence for the construct validity of a measure. For example, the Community Integration Questionnaire (CIQ) has 15 items that ask a person about their everyday activities at home, in their local community, and in education or work settings Willer et al. (1993). Although we cannot see or measure community integration directly (hence the name latent variable), in the same way that we can measure height, weight or blood pressure, the assumption is that the construct is nonetheless real and is reflected in the scores on the 15 items of the CIQ. Using factor analysis researchers have demonstrated that the 15 items of the CIQ form three clusters or factors representing *home integration, community integration* and *productive activity* (Hirsh et al., 2011). This correspondence between the factors or item groupings underpinning the CIQ and the notions about community integration espoused by the test authors is offered as support for its construct validity.

Another method for demonstrating construct validity derives from the method of convergent/discriminant validity (Bowling, 2000). Convergent validity requires the scale to 'correlate with related variables' and discriminant validity requires the scale 'not to correlate with dissimilar variables'. Although this seems like obvious common sense it is an important point and gives an indication that measuring outcome is based on theory and an understanding how a measurement tool should behave if it is valid. Finally, it is important to note that the construct validation of a measure is never completed. It is a cumulative process that draws evidence from a wide range of methods all of which shed some light on the relationship between the measure and the construct underpinning it.

Responsiveness

A key aspect of any clinical measure is that scores on the measure change when the patient's actual clinical condition changes – and in the same direction. This is known as responsiveness. It is the other side of the coin from test–retest reliability that we discussed earlier. We want a measure on which the scores are relatively stable over short periods of time when the person's state or condition is stable (i.e. reliability) and we want a measure that is responsive to quite small changes in the same state or condition. It is very much the same as your bathroom scales. You want a set of scales that give the same weight when your weight is stable, hopefully for most of the year, but you also need them to tell you as soon as you start putting on extra weight e.g. soon after feasts and festivities.

Responsiveness is usually tested by administering the same measure on two occasions when a change in condition is considered highly probable. So, for example, we might administer a QoL questionnaire before and after patients went on a drug treatment known to be highly effective at relieving a certain condition. Or we might test the responsiveness of a measure of activity and participation by administering it at admission and discharge from inpatient rehabilitation. Ideally when we measure responsiveness in this way we will also have other measures of the changes in patients to corroborate that the new measure is responsive to real changes in the condition. Importantly, responsiveness is always linked to the unit of measurement, the level of data collected, the range of values and the minimal detectable change for a particular scale.

Responsiveness is measured by two principle methods: anchor-based and distribution-based approaches. Anchor-based approaches use two end-points for classification, usually presented in a visual analogue scale. The two end-points could be, the very best health scenario (perfect health, no pain) and the very worst scenario (death, worst imaginable pain). Responsiveness is the distance moved between these two anchor points. The distribution-based approach does not use an anchor for defining meaningful change. Distribution approaches estimate the amount of error and variation in the concepts being measured in relation to the size of the sample. If large group differences exist between baseline and follow-up for a sample of patients then a reasonable measure should detect this change. If the group difference is small then only a particularly responsive measure will detect this (Adams et al., 2010). This information is useful to us as health professionals as we want to use a measure with our patient that is going to detect change if change is occurring. It is therefore relevant to choose outcome measures that can detect changes in our patient groups and as clinicians and researchers we need to look to evidence of straightforward comparative studies of different outcomes over time to help us decide which may be the most appropriate outcome measure to use.

Responsiveness is usually measured by any one of a number of statistics including the effect size, the standardised response mean and the responsiveness index. Unfortunately, there are at least three different formulas that can be used just for calculating an effect size and no real consensus on which index is the best to use to most accurately reflect responsiveness (Middel and van Sonderen, 2002). To complicate matters even further there is some evidence from rehabilitation that these different indexes of responsiveness can give quite different impressions of the responsiveness of a particular measure (Kuijer et al., 2005). To give an illustration of this, research into hip replacement surgery outcomes suggests that these indexes can differ quite substantially (Wright and Young, 1997) whereas, in lumbar spine surgery each index produced similar results (Stucki et al., 1995). Responsiveness is also context and population specific. So a measure that is responsive with one particular diagnostic group of patients may not be as responsive with another diagnostic group. It is relevant to understand what type of measure you choose to use as, although disease- or diagnostic-specific scales are reported as being more responsive than generic scales (Wright and Young, 1997), individualized patient preference scales (i.e. those scales that concentrate on specific concerns of individual patients) have been reported as the most responsive of all (Tugwell et al., 1994). If you are trying to decide exactly which outcome measures to use it may be wise to pick two; one generic measure that can capture broader functional or participation issues and one disease-specific measure.

It is also useful to understand what might contribute to score changes for your patients. When patients complete outcome measures over time the way that they rate their ability can be affected by their self-appraisal of their performance or status changing over the course of their disease (Rapkin and Schwartz, 2004) and changes in their habituation and coping mechanisms (Schwartz and Rapkin, 2004). This is particularly relevant for people with long-term conditions where patients may develop more effective coping mechanisms over time but still experience the same level of disability.

Lastly, there is little information that identifies what difference in outcome is required to represent a meaningful change on a scale. So just recording figures and numbers is not particularly informative for patients or clinicians unless that figure or number has a real meaning. In rehabilitation it tends to be that patient and clinician ratings of change remain the 'gold standard'. This rating can be done quite simply by asking patients if they feel that any change is relevant or important for them. Using a simple visual analogue scale can give you this information. Although this might be confusing for non-statisticians it is probably a reflection of an evolving and developing part of rehabilitation science where some uncertainties remain. From a practical perspective it suggests that when you are considering a measure to use in clinical practice be sure to look for more than a single research study in support of the responsiveness of your measure.

Recent advances in psychometrics

Psychometrics is a field that has developed rapidly aided greatly by the use of modern high speed computers and statistical software packages. Since the late 1960s Item Response Theory models have become increasingly influential and in rehabilitation the use of Rasch analysis in particular is competing with traditional psychometric approaches based on Classical Test Theory (DeVellis, 2006; Pallant and Tennant, 2007). However, the issues are technical and go well beyond the intended scope of this text. Interested readers are referred elsewhere for more information on this exciting and flourishing area (Tennant and Conaghan, 2007).

5.3   Applying outcome measures in clinical practice

Using 'indicators'

When working clinically it can be tempting to try and measure as much as possible so that we can understand exactly what is (and is not) changing for our patients. However, in practice we rarely have the time to measure and interpret everything and it can place unnecessary burden on our patients. This is where the concept of using outcome measures as 'indicators' of broader concepts can be useful. Adams and colleagues illustrated a working example of this. Their study examined the practicality of using a very quick and time efficient power hand grip measure as an indicator of broader aspects of function such as hand pain, dexterity and self-reported hand function for people with rheumatoid arthritis (Adams et al., 2004). In practice, if we have simple, brief measures that demonstrate a strong correlation with other areas of function then we can make some assumptions about our patients' wider performance. For example, the analysis of various outcome measures (clinician-rated functional grip ability and dexterity, self- reported upper limb function and hand joint deformity) used in determining upper limb functional performance in early rheumatoid arthritis, showed that power hand grip correlated very strongly with overall upper limb ability and self-report functional ability – and could therefore be used confidently as an indicator of broader performance in people with early rheumatoid arthritis affecting their hands. There is usually no single variable that can capture everything we would like to measure clinically so having an indicator that has been shown to correlate well with certain important outcomes can save time and effort and offer broader insight into patient performance and status without excessive testing and measuring.

Normative comparison values

When considering a patient's score on a measure we are usually interested to see whether their score has gone up, down or stayed the same over a period of time. However, it can also be informative to compare their performance to that of other people of a similar age, gender, education, ethnicity or disease status. For example, a score below 24 on the Mini-Mental Status Examination is often used as a cut-off score indicating possible cognitive impairment (Folstein et al., 1975). This is based on the idea that nearly all adults with intact cognitive abilities can score 24 or higher on this brief screening test. As health professionals when we review an individual patient's status and progress it is often useful to have reference or normative scores available so that comparisons can be made with expected values. Although extensive data on normative or reference values exist in certain specialities such as neuropsychology, in much of rehabilitation this kind of normative information is often limited or difficult to locate, as the work of developing and compiling normative data is still ongoing. However, Backman and her team have provided an excellent example of how this can be done for a clinical hand assessment. The Arthritis Hand Function Test (Backman et al., 1991) was developed as a tool that incorporates excellent reference ranges of performance against other patients with mild, moderate and severe arthritis affecting their hands. In using and interpreting this tool patients and clinicians are able to classify functional performance against age and gender norms for each part of the assessment and gain clearer insight about comparative performances.

The use of national / international core sets

In some areas of rehabilitation there now exist specialist interest groups and organizations who have worked to develop recommended core sets of outcome measures that should be included in every patient's assessment. If you are lucky enough to work within one of these speciality areas where work on developing core sets has already been done then take advantage of this. An example of where such collaboration with specialist groups has had an international impact is within rheumatology. The OMERACT initiative (http://www.intermed.med.uottawa.ca/research/omeract./) is an informal international group of patients, clinicians and academics that works to improve outcome measurement in rheumatology through a regular, interactive, consensus process. Such a process helps to ensure that what is recommended to be measured has been informed by patients, clinicians and academics. In this instance the group have been able to define what they agree to be measured as a 'core set of outcomes' for patients with rheumatoid arthritis around the world and to start developing a potential international database (Tugwell et al., 2007).

Scoring

It is essential when using any outcome measures in practice to fully understand the scoring procedure for any outcome measure you choose to adopt. Some measures have a complete manual that provides detailed instructions on administration, scoring and interpretation. Other measures are contained in the original journal articles where they were first published and may only have minimal information on administration and scoring. We suggest, before using any measure with patients for the first time, that you practise administering and scoring it – ideally on yourself and any kind colleagues who will oblige. Be aware that some scoring systems may even penalize patients for using equipment or receiving assistance from carers to complete daily tasks. The Health Assessment Questionnaire (HAQ) (Fries et al., 1980) is one such functional PROM. So if you are using the HAQ to record the functional ability of your patients and you have provided them with some assistive daily living equipment to make their life safer, easier and more independent they will receive lower scores indicating a worse outcome rather than higher scores on the HAQ. So be careful which PROMs you decide to use – particularly if these are going to be used as tools to review service provision and effectiveness of interventions.

Cultural relevance

An important issue in the use of any standardized questionnaire or rating scale is the extent to which that instrument can be considered relevant and appropriate for use with people of a particular culture (Geisinger, 1994). This issue is especially complex in practice because most rehabilitation measurement instruments have been developed in the USA or UK (Høegh and Høegh, 2009). For example the DASH (Disability of Arm, Shoulder and Hand) was developed in the USA in the 1990s to assess symptoms and functioning in people with upper limb impairments. Since then it has been adapted for use in Greek, Brazilian Portuguese, Armenian and Russian, Canadian French, Chinese, Italian, German and Swedish (Alotaibi, 2008). In health settings it is crucial that any self-report measure has been rigorously validated for use in a country or with members of a culture other than the one it was developed with initially.

Høegh and Høegh suggest that there are three important steps in trans-adapting (or translating and adapting) any health outcome measure for use across cultures: (1) linguistic translation, (2) cultural adaptation, and (3) item elimination or addition. The first stage involves translating the text of the measure (instructions, questions, response scale) into the other language. The second stage is concerned with ensuring that the concepts or constructs underpinning the measure have relevance and are meaningful within the culture or society concerned. The third step involves removing any items that 'do not work' and replacing them with more culturally relevant items. A key part of this adaptation process is known as *back translation*. This refers to a process whereby the original tool is first translated into the desired language (say Spanish) and a second 'blind' translator then translates the new Spanish version back into the original language (usually English). If the back translated version is almost identical to the original text then the process of translation is considered valid. Back translation is only one element in the complex process of trans-adaptation or cross-cultural validation of a tool or measure. Fortunately, guidelines exist to assist clinicians and researchers who intend to adapt an existing measure for use in other cultures (Beaton et al., 2000; Geisinger, 1994).

Personal impact for patients

An ongoing challenge for people who design outcome measures and those who use them is that not all questions are relevant or pertinent to each individual. This then results in an outcome measure that has potentially limited applicability for each patient. For example, someone with ankylosing spondylitis may be given the widely used HAQ (Fries et al., 1980) to review their self-reported functional ability. Questions are asked about set situations that do not necessarily weigh the impact of any functional disability. For instance, an individual may not be able to take a bath (one of the set questions on the HAQ), but for them this has less impact if they are able to use a shower and are perfectly happy with this. However, there is no scope within the remit of the measure to record how much any such limitation matters to the individual. Recognition that this measure provided information that was factually correct but limited, led to the development of the Personal Impact Health Assessment Questionnaire (PI-HAQ) (Hewlett et al., 2002). This development from the original HAQ now measures the individual values for functions, which can then be used to weight the level of an individual patient's functional loss and calculate the personal impact of disability.

A related example of this issue is that relatively few questionnaires ask patients about their satisfaction with their abilities. For example, the Michigan Hand Outcomes Questionnaire (Chung et al., 1998) asks patients to rate their hand strength, function and movement but also how satisfied they are with this level of performance. This is another positive way to try and ensure that the relevance of any limitation or disability is seen in the context of how important it is to the patient.

5.4 Conclusion

The use of PROMs for clinical practice, service evaluation and research is becoming an essential and often required aspect of modern rehabilitation. The involvement of rehabilitation consumers in deciding what to measure and in developing valid measures is now a routine part of constructing PROMs. There is also an increasingly sophisticated array of psychometric techniques to ensure these measures are robust statistically. Moreover, the ICF provides a comprehensive and conceptually rich framework for applying PROMs in a rehabilitation context. At the same time the use of PROMs in rehabilitation demands the same degree of professional skill, judgement and sensitivity as any other clinical activity. The routine use of PROMs needs to be an integral part of a reflective approach to clinical practice – we always need to be careful that it does not become a sterile exercise in number crunching.

Additional resources

Bowling, A. (2005). *Measuring Health: A Review of Quality of Life Measurement Scales (3rd edn)*. Maidenhead: Open University Press.

Finch, E., Brooks, D., Stratford, P. W. and Mayo, N., E. (2002). *Physical Rehabilitation Outcome Measures: A Guide to enhanced Clinical Decision Making (2nd edn)*. Ottowa: Canadian Physiotherapy Association.

Streiner, D. L. and Norman, G. R. (2008). *Health Measurement Scales: A Practical Guide to their Development and Use (4th edn)*. Oxford: Oxford University Press.

Tate, R. L. (2010). *A compendium of Tests, Scales And Questionnaires: The Practitioners Guide to Measuring Outcomes after Brain Impairment*. Hove: Psychology Press.

Wade, D. T. (1991). *Measurement in Neurological Rehabilitation*. Oxford: Oxford University Press.

References

Adams, J., Burridge, J., Mullee, M., Hammond, A. and Cooper, C. (2004). Correlation between upper limb functional ability and structural hand impairment in an early rheumatoid population. *Clinical Rehabilitation*, *18*, 405–413.

Adams, J., Bradley, S. and Chapman, J. (2009). Literacy levels required to complete patient reported outcome measures in rheumatology. *Annals of the Rheumatic Diseases*, *68*(3), 771.

Adams, J., Mullee, M., Burridge, J., Hammond, A. and Cooper, C. (2010). The responsiveness of self-report and therapist rated upper limb structural impairment and functional outcome measures in early rheumatoid arthritis. *Arthritis Care and Research*, *62*(2), 274–278.

Alotaibi, N. (2008). The cross-cultural adaptation of the disability of arm, shoulder and hand (DASH): a systematic review. *Occupational Therapy International*, *15*(3), 178–190.

Anastasi, A. and Urbina, S. (1997). *Psychological Testing*. Upper Saddle River, NJ: Prentice-Hall Inc.

Backman, C., Mackie, H. and Harris, J. (1991). Arthritis Hand Function Test: development of a standardised assessment tool. *The Occupational Therapy Journal of Research*, *11*(4), 245–255.

Barnes, M. and Ward, A. (2000). *Textbook of Rehabilitation Medicine*. Oxford: Oxford University Press.

Beaton, D., Bombardier, C., Guillemin, F. and Ferraz, M. (2000). Guidelines for the process of cross-cultural adaptation of self-report measures. *Spine*, *25*(24), 3186–3189.

Beaton, D., Wright, J., Katz, J. and Upper Extremity Group. (2005). Development of the QuickDASH: comparison of three item-reduction approaches. *Journal of Bone Joint Surgery 87*, 1038–1046.

Bowling, A. (2000). *Measuring Disease (2nd Edition)*. Buckingham: Open University Press.

Bowling, A. (2005). *Measuring Health: A Review of Quality of Life Measurement Scales. (3rd edn)*. Maidenhead: Open University Press.

Calman, K. C. (1984). Quality of life in cancer patients - an hypothesis. *Journal of Medical Ethics*, *10*, 124–127.

Chesson, R., Macleod, M. and Massie, S. (1996). Outcome measures in therapy departments in Scotland. *Physiotherapy*, *82*(12), 673–679.

Chung, K. C., Pillsbury , M. S., Walters, M. R., Hayward, R. A. and Arbor, A. (1998). Reliability and validity testing of the Michigan Hand Outcomes Questionnaire. *The Journal of Hand Surgery*, *23A*(4), 575–587.

Copeland, J., Taylor, W. and Dean, S. (2008). Factors influencing the use of outcome measures for patients wth low back pain: a survey of New Zealand physical therapists. *Physical Therapy*, *88*(12), 1492–1505.

Dellhag, B. and Bjelle, A. (1995). A grip ability test for use in rheumatology practice. *The Journal of Rheumatology*, *22*(8), 1559–1565.

DeVellis, R. (2006). Classical Test Theory. *Medical Care*, *44*(11), s50–s59.

Devinsky, O., Vickrey, B.G., Cramer, J., Perrine, K., Hermann, B., Meador, K. and Hays, R.D. (1995). Development of the Quality of Life in Epilepsy Inventory. *Epilepsia*, *36*(11), 1089–1104.

Division of Mental Health and Prevention of Substance Abuse, World Health Organization. (1997). *WHOQOL - Measuring Quality of Life*. Geneva: World Health Organization.

Fayers, P. M. and Machin, D. (2007). *Quality of Life: The Assessment, Analysis and Interpretation of Patient-Reported Outcomes*. Chichester: John Wiley and Sons.

Finch, E., Brooks, D., Stratford, P. and Mayo, N. (2002). *Physical Rehabilitation Outcome Measures: A Guide to Enhanced Clinical Decision Making (2nd edn)*. Ottawa: Canadian Physiotherapy Association.

Folstein, M. F., Folstein, S. E. and McHugh, P. R. (1975). "Mini-Mental State": A practical method for grading the cognitive state of patients for the clinician. *Journal of Psychiatric Research*, *12*, 189–198.

Fries, J., Spitz, P., Kraines, R. and Holman, H. (1980). Measurement of patient outcome in arthritis. *Arthritis and Rheumatism*, *23*(2), 137–145.

Geisinger, K. (1994). Cross-cultural normative assessment: Translation and adaptation issues influencing the normative interpretation of assessment instruments. *Psychological Assessment*, *6*(4), 304–312.

Greenhalgh, J. (2009). The applications of PROs in clinical practice: what are they, do they work, and why? *Quality of Life Research*, *18*, 115–123.

Hearn, J. and Higginson, I. J. (1999). Development and validation of a core outcome measure for palliative care: the Palliative Care Outcome Scale *Quality in Health Care*, *8*, 219–217.

Hewlett, S., Smith, A. and Kirwan, J. (2002). Extended report: measuring the meaning of disability in rheumatoid arthritis: the Personal Impact Health Assessment Questionnaire (PI HAQ). *Annals of the Rheumatic Diseases*, *61*, 986–993.

Hirsh, A., Braden, A., Craggs, J. and Jensen, M. (2011). Psychometric properties of the Community Integration Questionnaire in a heterogeneous sample of adults with physical disability. *Archives of Physical Medicine and Rehabilitation*, *92*, 1602–1610.

Høegh, M. and Høegh, S. (2009). Trans-adapting outcome measures in rehabilitation: cross-cultural issues. *Neuropsychological Rehabilitation*, *19*(6), 955–970.

Hudak, P. L., Amadio, P. C. and Bombardier, C. (1996). Development of an upper extremity outcome measure: the DASH (Disabilities of the Arm, Shoulder and Hand). *American Journal of Industrial Medicine*, *29*, 602–608.

Huijbregts, M., Myers, A., Kay, T. and Gavin, T. (2002). Systematic outcome measurement in clinical practice: Challenges experienced by physiotherapists. *Physiotherapy Canada*, *54*(1), 25–36.

Hush, J.M., Refshauge, K.M., Sullivan, G., DeSouza, L. and McAuley, J.H. (2010). Do numerical rating scales and the Roland-Morris Disability Questionnaire capture changes that are meaningful to patients with persistent back pain? *Clinical Rehabilitation*, *24*, 648–657.

Jette, D., Halbert, J., Iverson, C., Miceli, E. and Shah, P. (2009). Use of standardised outcome measures in physical therapist practice: Perceptions and applications. *Physical Therapy*, *89*(2), 125–135.

Kolakowsky-Hayner, S., Kreutzer, J. and Miner, D. (2000). Validation of the service obstacles scale for the traumatic brain injury population. *Neurorehabilitation*, *14*, 151–158.

Kuijer, W., Brouwer, S., Dijkstra, P., Jorritsma, W., Groothof, J. and Geertzen, J. (2005). Responsiveness of the Roland Morris Disability Questionnaire: consequences of using different external criteria. *Clinical Rehabilitation, 19*, 488–495.

Leplege, A. and Hunt, S. (1997). The problem of quality of life in medicine. *Journal of the American Medical Association, 278*(1), 47–50.

Marshall, S., Haywood, K. and Fitzpatrick, R. (2005). *Patient Involvement and Collaboration in Shared Decision-Making: A Structured Review to inform Chronic Disease Management. Report from the Patient-reported Health Instruments Group to the Department of Health.* Oxford: National Centre for Health Outcomes at the University of Oxford.

Marwitz, J. and Kreutzer, J. (1996). *The Service Obstacles Scale (SOS).* Richmond, VA: Virginia Commonwealth University.

Meenan, R. (1982). The AIMS approach to health status measurement: conceptual background and measurement properties. *The Journal of Rheumatology, 9*(5), 785–788.

Michell, J. (1990). *An Introduction to the Logic of Psychological Measurement.* Hillsdale, NJ: Lawrence Erlbaum Associates.

Michell, J. (2000). Normal science, pathological science and psychometrics. *Theory and Psychology, 10*(5), 639–667.

Middel, B. and van Sonderen, E. (2002). Statistical significant change versus relevant or important change in (quasi) experimental design: some conceptual and methodological problems in estimating magnitude of intervention-related change in health services research. *International Journal of Integrated Care, 2*, 1–17.

Nothnagl, T., Andel, I., Sautner, J., Leder, S., Bogdan, M., Maktari, A. and Leeb, B. F. (2005). Improvement and deterioration of rheumatoid arthritis: the patient's persepctive. *Annals of the Rheumatic Diseases, 64*(S111), 182.

Nunnally, J. and Bernstein, I. (1994). *Psychometric Theory (3rd edn).* New York: McGraw-Hill Inc.

Pallant, J. and Tennant, A. (2007). An introduction to the Rasch measurement model: an example using the Hospital Anxiety and Depression Scale (HADS). *British Journal of Clinical Psychology, 46*(1), 1–18.

Prevoo, M. (1995). Modified disease activity scores that include twenty-eight joint counts. Development and validation of patients with rheumatoid arthritis. *Arthritis and Rheumatism, 38*, 44–48.

Quality Metric. (n.d.) *SF HealthSurveys.* Lincoln RI: Quality Metric. www.qualitymetric.com/ WhatWeDo/GenericHealthSurveys/tabid/184/Default.aspx?gclid=CO3FkPyI66wCFQUht Aod6S3JNg (accessed 5 December 2011).

Rapkin, B. and Schwartz, C. (2004). Toward a theoretical model of quality-of-life appraisal:Implications of findings from studies of response shift. *Health and Quality of Life Outcomes, 2*, 14.

Rothwell, A., Sinnott, A., Mohammed, K., Dunn, J. and Sinclair, S. (2003). Upper limb surgery for tetraplegia: a 10-year re-review of hand function. *The Journal of Hand Surgery, 28a*(3), 489–495.

Sakakibara, B., Miller, W., Orenczuk, S. and Wolfe, D. (2009). A systematic review of depression and anxiety measures used with individuals with spinal cord in jury. *Spinal Cord, 47*(12), 841–851.

Salaffi, F., Filipucci, Gasparinin, S., Gutierrez, Savic, V., Ciapetti, A. and Grassi, W. (2005). Self-reported twenty eight joint counts in rheumatoid arthritis: comparison with physician's joint count. *Annals of the Rheumatic Diseases, 64*(S111), 205.

Schwartz, C. and Rapkin, B. (2004). Reconsidering the psychometrics of quality of life assessment in light of response shift and appraisal. *Health and Quality of Life Outcomes*, 2, 16.

Siegert, R.J., Patten, M. and Walkey, F. (1987). Development of a brief Social Support Questionnaire. *New Zealand Journal of Psychology*, 16, 79–83.

Siegert, R.J., Walkey, F. and Turner-Stokes, L. (2009). An examination of the factor structure of the Beck Depression Inventory-II in a neurorehabilitation inpatient sample. *Journal of the International Neuropsychological Society*, 15, 142–147.

Siegert, R.J., Gao Wei, Walkey, F. H., and Higginson, I. J. (2010). Psychological well-being and quality of care: A factor-analytic examination of the Palliative Care Outcome Scale (POS). *Journal of Pain and Symptom Management*, 40 (1), 67-74.

Siegert, R.J., Tennant, A. and Turner-Stokes, L. (2010). Rasch analysis of the Beck Depression Inventory-II in a neurological rehabilitation sample. *Disability and Rehabilitation*, 32(1), 8–17.

Sinnott, K., Dunn, J. and Rothwell, A. (2004). Use of the ICF conceptual framework to interpret hand function outcomes following tendon transfer for tetraplegia. *Spinal Cord*, 42, 396–400.

Sinnott, K., Brander, P., Siegert, R., Rothwell, A. and DeJong, G. (2009). Life impacts following reconstructive hand surgery for tetraplegia. *Topics in Spinal Cord Injury*, 15, 90–97.

Skinner, A. and Turner-Stokes, L. (2006). The use of standardised outcome measures in rehabilitation centres in the UK. *Clinical Rehabilitation*, 20, 609–615.

Spiegel, T. M., Spiegel, J. S. and Paulus, H. E. (1987). The Joint Alignment and Motion Scale: a simple measure of joint deformity in patients with rheumatoid arthritis. *The Journal of Rheumatology*, 145, 887–892.

Stamm, T., van der Giesen, F., Thorstensson, C., Steen, E., Birrell, F., Bauernfeind, B. and Kloppenburg, M. (2009). Patient perspective of hand osteoarthritis in relation to concepts covered by instruments measuring functioning: a qualitative European multicentre study, *Annals of the Rheumatic Diseases*, 68, 1453–1460.

Streiner, D. and Norman, G. (2008). *Health Measurement Scales (4th edn)*. Oxford: Oxford University Press.

Streiner, D.L. (2003). Starting at the beginning: an introduction to coefficient alpha and internal consistency. *Journal of Personality Assessment*, 80(1), 99–103.

Stucki, G., Stucki, S., Bruhlmann, Maus, S. and Michel, B. (1995). Comparison of the validity and reliability of self-reported articular indices. *British Journal of Rheumatology*, 34, 760–766.

Taylor, W., Myers, J., Simpson, R., McPherson, K. and Weatherall, M. (2004). Quality of life of people with rheumatoid arthritis as measured by the World Health Organization Quality of Life Instrument, Short Form (WHOQOL-BREF): score distributions and psychometric properties. *Arthritis and Rheumatism (Arthritis Care and Research)*, 51(3), 350–357.

Teasdale, G. and Jennett, B. (1974). Assessment of coma and impaired consciousness. *The Lancet*, 304(7872), 81–84.

Tennant, A. and Conaghan, P. (2007). The Rasch measurement model in rheumatology: what is it and why use it? When should it be applied, and what should one look for in a Rasch paper? *Arthritis Care and Research*, 57(8), 1358–1362.

Tugwell, P., Boers, M., Baker, P., Wells, G. and Sinder, J. (1994). Endpoints in rheumatoid arthritis. *Journal of Rheumatology*, 21(S42), 2–8.

Tugwell, P., Boers, M., Brooks, P., Simon, L., Strand, V. and Idzerda, L. (2007). OMERACT: an international initiative to improve outcome measurement in rheumatology. *Trials*, 8(1), 38.

Turner-Stokes, L., Nyein, K., Turner-Stokes, T., Gatehouse, C. (1999). The UK FIM + FAM: development and evaluation. *Clinical Rehabilitation*, 13, 277-287.

Tyson, S. (2009). The psychometric properties and clinical utility of measures of walking and mobility in neurological conditions: a systematic review. *Clinical Rehabilitation, 23*(11), 1018–1033.

US Department of Health and Human Services Food and Drug Administration. (2009). *Guidance for Industry - Patient-Reported Outcome Measures: Use in Medical Product Development to Support Labeling Claims.* Silver Spring, MD: US Food and Drug Administration. http://www.fda.gov/downloads/Drugs/GuidanceCompliance%20Regulatory Information/Guidances/UCM193282 (accessed on 5 December 2011).

Valderas, J., Kotzeva, A., Espallargues, M., Guyatt, G., Ferrans, C., Halyard, M. and Alonso, J. (2008). The impact of measuring patient-reported outcomes in clinical practice: a systematic review of the literature. *Quality of Life Research, 17*, 179–193.

Wade, D. (1991). *Measurement in Neurological Rehabilitation.* Oxford: Oxford University Press.

Wade, D. (2003). Outcome measures for clinical rehabilitation trials: impairment, function, quality of life, or value? *American Journal of Physical Medicine and Rehabilitation, 82* (Supplement), S26–S31.

Whalley, K. and Adams, J. (2009). The longitudinal validity of the quick and full version of the Disability of the Arm Shoulder and Hand Questionnaire in musculoskeletal hand out patients. *Journal of Hand Therapy, 14*(1), 22–25.

Willer, B., Rosenthal, M., Kreutzer, J.S., Gordon, W.A., Rempel, R. (1993). Assessment of community integration following rehabilitation for traumatic brain injury. *The Journal of Head Trauma Rehabilitation, 8* (2), 75-87.

World Health Organization. (2001). *ICF: International Classification of Functioning, Disability and Health.* Geneva: WHOs.

Wright, J. G. and Young, N. L. (1997). A comparison of different indices of responsiveness. *Journal of Clinical Epidemiology, 50*(3), 239–246.

Zigmond, A. and Snaith, R. (1983). The Hospital Anxiety and Depression Scale. *Acta Psychiatrica Scandinavia, 67*, 361–370.

Zuercher, M., Ummenhofer, W., Baltussen, A. and Walder, B. (2009). The use of the Glasgow Coma Scale in injury assessment: a critical review. *Brain Injury, 23*(5), 371–384.

Chapter 6

The person in context

Julie Pryor[1] *and Sarah G. Dean*[2]

[1]*Director of the Rehabilitation Nursing Research & Development Unit, Royal Rehabilitation Centre, Sydney and Associate Professor, Rehabilitation and Aged Care, Flinders University, Adelaide, Australia;* [2]*Senior Lecturer in Health Services Research, University of Exeter Medical School, United Kingdom*

6.1 Introduction

This is the last of the five core themes of rehabilitation that we wish to present in this book. The theme is about how rehabilitation in the 21st Century is charged with understanding the patient who is taking part in rehabilitation and their context, thereby placing this person at the centre of rehabilitation. Although 'the person in context' is the final theme of the textbook, it has not been placed last because it has least status; instead this theme is the culmination of the preceding chapters and is perhaps the most important of all the themes we have presented.

This chapter will cover a number of issues and begins with identifying who are the stakeholders in rehabilitation. It goes on to provide some key definitions and to examine what is meant by 'person' and 'personhood', 'person-centredness' as well as the personal factors domain of the ICF (World Health Organization (WHO), 2001). We then consider in some detail, the individual and collective experiences of rehabilitation and how rehabilitation following acquired disability might be regarded as a personal journey; examining also the work and participation aspects of 'doing' rehabilitation. We briefly re-visit patient priorities and goal setting, considering their life goals as opposed to treatment goals, and how rehabilitation challenges a person's view of their life and what they are capable of. Our discussion then extends to cover some broader environmental contextual issues: the importance of placing the person in their family context and how we might involve families in rehabilitation; the role of clinical services with some examples to show how clinical pathways or different types of service arrangements can affect rehabilitation provision for an individual person. We also touch briefly upon some of the wider contextual issues that affect how rehabilitation might be experienced by an individual, such as the physical

Interprofessional Rehabilitation: A Person-Centred Approach, First Edition.
Edited by Sarah G. Dean, Richard J. Siegert and William J. Taylor.
© 2012 John Wiley & Sons, Ltd. Published 2012 by John Wiley & Sons, Ltd.

environment, social and cultural factors, as well as the impact of different types of healthcare policy and funding. However, we do not attempt comprehensive coverage of these broader contextual issues rather offering some illustrative examples that relate specifically to rehabilitation practice.

In Section 6.9 we move away from some of the theoretical and service perspectives and instead provide some challenges for the reader to work through. We ask the reader to consider their own personhood, to examine what they bring to the rehabilitation process and how they might develop their skills of focusing on the individual at the centre of rehabilitation. We also provide a few examples of how person-centred healthcare is being implemented at organizational levels and in applied healthcare research. The chapter ends with a summary of whether we think it is possible to do person-centred rehabilitation.

6.2   Who are the stakeholders in rehabilitation?

Rehabilitation is a complex healthcare intervention (Cameron, 2010; Wade, 2005) that uses interventions that range from a macro to a micro level (Whyte and Hart, 2003). At the macro level, the built environment can shape team functioning and affect patient outcomes (Clarke, 2010; Pryor, 2008). At the micro level, positioning of an upper limb can influence patient outcomes. The multiplicity of levels of interventions and the many interactions between them make rehabilitation a complex and incompletely understood science, the outcomes of which are of interest to a range of stakeholders.

Although the person with disability is acknowledged as the one who can ultimately determine whether rehabilitation works or not (Cameron, 2010), others too have an interest in the outcomes of rehabilitation. At the family level, the outcomes of an individual's rehabilitation may influence interpersonal relationships, social and domestic roles as well as the economy of the family unit. At the community level, the outcomes of an individual's rehabilitation may impact on sporting teams, recreation groups, church congregations or political activities. As such, society as a whole has an interest in the outcomes of rehabilitation (DeJong et al., 2004), with reduction in disability and improvement in participation in life being the ultimate aims of rehabilitation at policy level (D'Alisa et al., 2005).

With so many stakeholders it is easy to lose sight of the individuals who are the reason for the existence of rehabilitation services. Although few would say that the person who is the patient is not central to the processes of rehabilitation, it is seldom recognized that the perspectives of staff and patients are not always the same. Therefore the focus of this chapter is to examine rehabilitation from the perspective of people experiencing disability. It explores human responses to acquired disability and patients' experiences of rehabilitation service delivery. This leads the reader to think about definitions and meanings of words relating to the 'person in context'.

6.3   Key terms

Terms that are central to consideration of the 'person in context' are 'person' and 'personhood', 'person-centredness' and 'personal factors' as well as 'patient-centredness' and 'personalization'.

Person and personhood

It is not easy to define what makes a human being a person or what the key characteristics are that can be used to describe personhood. This may be why these terms are not a feature of the rehabilitation literature. Web dictionary definitions are rather disappointing, with person defined as 'a human being ... man, woman or child' as distinguished from an animal or thing (dictionary.com, n.d.). Elaborations such as, 'the actual self or individual personality of a human being' (dictionary.com, n.d.) are slightly more helpful. Similarly, definitions of personhood as simply 'the state or fact of being a person' (dictionary.com, n.d.) are limited. The addition of a reference to 'qualities that confer distinct individuality' (The free dictionary.com, n.d.), however, indicates the uniqueness of each person. So what does being a person entail?

One way to answer this question is to examine the foundation stones of personhood. These might be considered to be the fundamental or primary 'goods' of life that are sought for their own sake, namely: life, knowledge, excellence, agency, inner peace, relatedness, community, spirituality, happiness and creativity (Siegert et al., 2007). According to Siegert et al. (2007, p. 1608), these primary goods are 'actions, states of affairs, personal characteristics, experiences and states of mind that are viewed as intrinsically beneficial to human beings' and as such we have called them the foundation stones of personhood. This 'personhood' also needs to be sustained, or supported. Siegert and colleagues (2010) regard the metaphor of a scaffold as 'helpful for people with disabilities' because the extent and strength of the scaffold equates to the intensity of support required, whereas the duration that a scaffold is in place relates to the time over which support is required. This scaffolding might comprise the five human rights-related goods of: personal freedom, material substance, personal security, elemental equality and social recognition (Siegert et al., 2010). Alternatively, Seligman's (2011) five elements of human well-being (positive emotion, engagement, meaning, accomplishment and positive relationships) could be used as scaffolding. Despite individual differences and idiosyncrasies, we all need some degree of scaffolding (Siegert et al., 2010). The list of environmental factors in the ICF (WHO, 2001) contains many examples of scaffolding. When seen as part of a system, the family and/or community are important aspects of an individual's scaffolding, as described in this mother's story:

> 'A few very short years ago I lost my son when his bodily form was occupied by the symptoms of an unforgiving disease. As the health care professionals treated the disease, family and friends transformed into supporters of his rehabilitation. A primary aspect of my role was preserving his integrity as a person, by maintaining continuity of his body and his self. To do this I maintained contact with the person who was my son to ensure that his

worldview was central to decisions made about him. Handing these responsibilities over to him was a difficult but necessary next step for him to be his own person' (Anon).

Importantly, personhood is not static. It has temporal, experiential and perhaps spatial considerations, as indicated by Kirschner (1997, p. 93) who asks 'who is this person known as Michael Martin?', it could be that Michael is the person who, prior to his head injury, had discussed with his wife some of his wishes about whether or not he would want to receive life sustaining treatment in the event of a major injury. However, Michael is also the person in the present, so Kirschner goes on to ask 'or is Michael Martin the man with an extensive head injury who is conscious, in no discernible distress, not terminally ill, and seemingly to indicate that he would prefer to live?' (Kirschner, 1997, p. 93). This example shows how difficult it can be to make a decision about something that one has yet to experience and equally how difficult it is to make decisions about another's care and future (and thus their personhood).

In contemplating personhood and what it is to be a person, it is worth considering if a human being can be something other than a person and whether it is possible to be a non-person. The 2006 United Nations Convention on the Rights of Persons with Disabilities suggests a way forward for addressing these difficult concepts; it notes that 'persons with disabilities are still primarily viewed as "objects" of welfare or medical treatment rather than "holders" of rights' (p. 4 cited in Siegert et al., 2010, p. 966). In contrast to this view of disability, Patston (2007) argues for more inclusive thinking around functional diversity, in which 'being' as well as 'doing' are valued. Seymour (1998, p. 20) says 'rehabilitation is a powerful agent for the ratification of particular types of bodies' suggesting rehabilitation services seem to favour the 'doing' and place less emphasis on the 'being' aspects of being human. Taking this point of view we can start to see that this type of service might not be very person-centred, a criticism of current rehabilitation, and why we are attempting to grapple with these issues as a theme for this book.

Person-centredness, patient-centredness and personalization

Much has been written about person-centred healthcare in the past decade, with many terms (such as 'patient-, client-, person-, individual-/-centred, -oriented, -focused, -directed') often being used interchangeably (Leplege et al., 2007, p. 1556). Although a consensus is yet to be reached about its meaning and implications (Leplege et al., 2007; Michie et al., 2003), the central tenet of person-centredness is 'respect for and integration of individual differences when delivering patient care' (Lauver et al., 2002, p. 248), with the critical characteristics being:

- understanding the patient as a unique person presenting with individual character-istics, needs, values, beliefs, and preferences;
- responding flexibly to patients' individual needs and preferences by selecting and delivering interventions that are mindful of, and responsive to, the patients' needs and preferences.

(Souraya et al., 2006, p. 118)

Bensing et al. (2000) argue that communication is the 'royal pathway' to patient-centredness because: (1) the patient is the expert in their experience of symptoms, which makes health care professionals dependent upon them; (2) patients have different preferences and diversity is the norm; and (3) it is more appropriate 'to strengthen patient's capabilities' for self-management of chronic conditions that medicine cannot cure. Characteristics of person-centred communication are: taking a biopsychosocial perspective; seeing the patient as a person; sharing power and responsibility; creating a therapeutic alliance and viewing ourselves as persons (Mead and Bower, 2000). These authors highlight the importance of communication and taking the patient's perspective, however, Michie and colleagues (2003) reviewed what was meant by 'patient-centredness' for people with chronic illness and took the additional step of determining whether it mattered. In their review of 30 studies of health professional communication they found two distinct types of 'patient-centredness', one whereby health professionals elicited and discussed patient beliefs and one whereby health professionals went a step further and 'activated' their patients. It was noted that good health outcomes were more likely to be associated with the latter type of patient-centredness suggesting that 'activation' or patient empowerment is what matters.

There is one other term to consider in this section: 'personalization' (see, Department of Health, 2008, http://webarchive.nationalarchives.gov.uk). This has been described as the new paradigm in social care for people with chronic conditions, reflecting the move towards self-directed support, self-assessment and co-production of care (Cornes, 2011) and we will be revisiting the 'personalization agenda' later in this chapter.

Personal factors

As we have discussed in Chapter 2 the personal factors are a less well-known component of ICF (WHO, 2001). They are one of two sets of contextual factors, the other being environmental factors. Both sets of contextual factors can act as enablers or barriers to functioning. Although not yet classified in the same way as the other components of the ICF, personal factors are an important part of the conceptual model and are described as 'the particular background of an individual's life and living, and comprise features of the individual that are not part of a health condition or health states' (WHO, 2001, p. 17). Examples of personal factors include age, gender, ethnicity, culture, psychological assets and education. Clinicians discover through their practice how differences in personal factors between patients influence the processes and outcomes of rehabilitation. This is because it is difficult to systematically explore the scope and contribution of personal factors to a person's functioning and disability without a classification system. The ICF has created the framework for this classification but to revisit our earlier discussion (in Chapter 2) the ICF has been criticized for its inability to clearly portray the dynamic process of disablement, both 'the "here and now" that happens when personal characteristics collide with socio-environmental ones' (Masala and Petretto, 2008, p. 1242) and what happens across time (but see

Duggan et al., 2008 for research attempting to incorporate the dynamic features of the ICF in their study of women with spinal cord injury). In the ICF 'there is no explicit acknowledgement that the person has both a past and a future'; the ICF does not take into account 'temporal factors such as the person's stage of life and illness'; nor does it take into account personal values and a person's own evaluation of their quality of life ((QoL), Wade and Halligan, 2003, p. 351). Most importantly the ICF, as a classification system, has yet to provide a mechanism for classifying personal strengths or assets that a person can bring to their rehabilitation; as an example, one such asset commonly recognized in the rehabilitation literature is motivation (see Chapter 2 for more about attempts to classify personal factors and see Chapter 4 for more about the motivational processes).

So although personal factors are integral to the conceptual model of the ICF they have yet to be fully classified. This is a current limitation of the ICF as personal factors are critical to the processes and outcomes of rehabilitation for individuals, with each patient bringing their unique tapestry of personal factors that interact with their health conditions and environmental factors to influence their functioning and disability. Through exploration and consideration of individual and collective experiences of acquired disability and rehabilitation, a little light can be shed on a few aspects of this rich tapestry of personal factors that an individual brings to their rehabilitation experience.

6.4   The lived experience of acquired disability

As a starting point it is interesting to consider what, and how much, we know about the people who experience disability and rehabilitation. The demographic characteristics of people who acquire disability are available nationally and in some instances globally. For example, the average age of the individuals with 362 new spinal cord injuries recorded by Australia's six spinal units in 2007–2008 was 45 years and 84% of those who were traumatically injured were males (Norton, 2010). Similar characteristics were noted by a 1988–2009 European adult spinal injury cohort study that recorded 28,489 spinal fractures/dislocations and spinal cord injuries; the average age was 44.5 years and 65% were male (Hasler et al., 2011).

Data about rehabilitation service utilization are also available. For example, the Australasian Rehabilitation Outcomes Centre (AROC) reports that 722 episodes of inpatient rehabilitation were provided for spinal cord dysfunction, 5,284 for stroke, and 28,553 for orthopaedic conditions in Australia in 2008 (Simmonds et al., 2009). In the UK physiotherapy services for the year 2003–2004 amounted to 4.3 million new episodes of care. These figures included, for example, 988,100 hospital referrals for trauma and orthopaedics and 37,500 for non-surgical neurology (Department of Health, 2004).

But what do rehabilitation clinicians *really* know about these people as individuals? When considering this question try taking into account what you know about your patients' values, attitudes and beliefs and how these inform their worldview.

Check how much you know about what they like to do and with whom; and what they plan or hope to be doing in the future. For example, clinicians might know that a patient named Janine is a 34-year-old female who has sustained a brain injury in a motor vehicle accident. She lives in a three-bedroom single-level house with four steps at the front door in a suburb on the outskirts of the city, with her husband Alvin and two primary school-aged sons. She is the daughter of Wendy and Peter, who live about an hour's drive away, closer to the centre of the city; Wendy and Peter both work full time. Alvin's parents live overseas with the rest of his extended family. Janine works part time during school hours at the local library. Alvin works afternoon shift in a local factory. Clinicians may not know that Janine: aspires to own a book-shop; looks forward to braiding the hair of a little girl; is very particular about her appearance, always paying close attention to her weight, diet and exercise; witnessed the sexual assault of her best friend at the age of 8; is frightened of the dark and every Wednesday secretly visits her disabled niece, who was institutionalized soon after birth. Information such as this constitutes personal factors that Janine would bring to her interactions with rehabilitation clinicians. Each personal factor has the potential to facilitate or act as a barrier to Janine's engagement with rehabilitation.

In a different example, Barrow's (2008) account of Anne's story illustrates the impact specific personal factors can play in the lives and rehabilitation journeys of individuals. Anne's experience of living with acquired aphasia (loss of ability to speak) was informed and shaped by the prevailing cultural 'narratives of disability (i.e. the "inner stories we live by")'; for her being aphasic meant she possessed limited competence and, because she was disabled, she was less than whole (Barrow, 2008, p. 30). She did not possess a frame of reference that enabled her to see other alternatives, and 'her life revolved around activities that would "make her better"' (Barrow, 2008, p. 30). There are a number of psychological models that can be used to describe this situation and how someone might change during their rehabilitation journey. One model of change is called the Trans-Theoretical Model (Prochaska et al., 1992) whereby people move from pre-contemplation to contemplating change before proceeding to preparation (action planning) and actual change (action), and finally maintenance of change. In Anne's example she is in the pre-contemplation stage of change, she is not in a place where an alternative 'life story' is even possible to contemplate.

With these examples we can see how the individual biographical and autobiographical accounts of disability and lived experience studies are valuable sources for understanding individual and collective experiences of acquired disability and rehabilitation. They help us to understand rehabilitation as a personal journey.

6.5 Rehabilitation as a personal journey of reconstruction or transformation of the self

Rehabilitation is commonly understood as a physical process and we discussed the key processes in Chapter 4. Less well recognized is that for many patients rehabilitation entails 'the holistic reconstruction of the 'self' (Siegert et al., 2007, p. 1609). The literature tends to use complex terminology such as 'reconstruction' or 'transformation' to denote the changes that occur for a person as they adapt and find a way of coping (or not) with their new circumstances. The following are a few examples of the many ways that a chronic condition can impose on a person's life: extreme shortness of breath can hinder walking to the mailbox or chatting with friends; the cost of medications can have an impact on the money available for recreational pursuits; and much time can be spent attending healthcare appointments. Balancing life and a chronic condition can be a daily struggle, with tensions between the desire to live a normal life and the constraints imposed by the condition (Jeon et al., 2010).

Reconstruction of the self therefore includes finding a new 'normalcy'. In a study by DeSanto-Madeya this involved 'focusing on the injured person's abilities' with the goal of having 'a productive and full life' despite the physical limitations of spinal cord injury (DeSanto-Madeya, 2006, p. 282). This redefinition of normalcy, which has also been noted by people with other disabling conditions, namely stroke, arthritis and chronic pain (McPherson et al., 2004), can mediate the experience of acquired disability. So for many rehabilitation patients, the primacy of maintaining the self is paramount, with the experience of personal identity reconstruction, or transformation of the self, not uncommon. Table 6.1 provides a selection of studies and theoretical viewpoints that can inform our understanding about the reconstruction of the self.

The reconstruction of personhood is also influenced by contextual factors (as defined in the ICF). Levack et al. (2010) highlighted where internal (personal factors) and external (environmental factors) resources facilitated this reconstruction. Similarly, context was shown to be important in the process of recapturing self-care after stroke and spinal cord injury in a study by Guidetti et al. (2009). In this study, the role of healthcare professionals in shaping context through creating expectations and helping patients to see possibilities is illuminated. Thus, a positive context is created for reconstruction of the self and, in relation to this positive reappraisal approach, the term 'transformation' is sometimes seen in the literature. This describes how patients learn to transform their lives, although the relationship between transformative learning and transformation in a more general sense is not yet clear. One suggestion is that the person incorporates acquired disability and its consequences in their biographical flow rather than allowing the acquired disability to create a situation of biographical attack and disruption (Faircloth et al., 2004). However, incorporation is far from a linear process, with Secrest and Thomas (1999, p. 240) finding that stroke survivors experience 'a sense of continuity that co-exists with discontinuity in the experience of self'.

Transformation of the self following acquired disability is also being linked with spirituality. For example, Faull and Hills (2006, p. 729) believe that 'the development of a resilient, intrinsic, spiritually based concept of self' may be crucial to rehabilitation outcomes. They suggest transformational coping is required for the development of such a self, with transformation 'allowing the retention of well-being by acknowledging disability as an opportunity for self-growth' (Faull and Hills, 2006, p.731). In line with this thinking, participants with adult-onset disability ($n = 6$) in a study by Schulz (2005) viewed disability as 'a catalyst for spiritual awakening' (p. 1291). Although

Table 6.1 Summarizing 'Reconstruction' and 'Transformation' of the self; a selection of examples from the rehabilitation literature.

Study details	Summary and comments
1 Morse (1997) 'Responding to threats to integrity of self'. Qualitative meta-synthesis, various chronic conditions and serious injury	Five stage theory of recovery and rehabilitation: 1 vigilance; 2 disruption: enduring to survive; 3 enduring to live: striving to regain self; 4 suffering: striving to restore self; 5 learning to live with the altered self Focus is on 'how the individual seeks self-comforting strategies to mediate the experience'. Work begins on the restoration of physical function in stage 3, but learning to live again as a whole person does not feature until stage 5. Personal factors that individuals might bring to their experience of recovery and rehabilitation were not explored
2 Leidy and Haase (1999) 'Preserving personal integrity'. Naturalistic qualitative study of 12 men and women with chronic obstructive pulmonary disease	Despite challenges in almost every aspect of their everyday life, these people actively sought a 'satisfying sense of wholeness'. This comprised a 'sense of effectiveness' and 'of connectedness' (p. 67). Central to the findings were the intrapersonal attribute of 'being able' to do things that indicated competence and the interpersonal attribute of 'being with' important others
3 Folkman and Moskowitz (2000) 'Attribution of meaning and positive reappraisal'. Theoretical paper	Transformation is explained as a gradual process triggered by a desire to mediate the experience of acquired disability. Mediating the challenges and difficulties associated with such experiences can be described as the work of coping. 'Coping' is classically defined as: 'constantly changing cognitive and behavioral efforts to manage specific external and/or internal demands that are appraised as taxing or exceeding the resources of the person' (Lazarus and Folkman, 1984, p. 141). Historically, the stress and coping literature has focused on the negative outcomes in the stress process, for example anger and depression. Noting that positive affect (mood) can co-exist with distress, challenges this thinking. Central to positive affect is the meaning an individual attributes to an event, situation or circumstance. Attribution of meaning is not a one-off event; reappraisal can change an initial 'glass half empty' to the more positive 'glass half full' view (Folkman and Moskowitz, 2000)
4 Kralik et al. (2005) 'Moving on or transition'. Qualitative study of six women with long-term illness	Moving on or transition involves seven interactive processes: 1 knowing one's response to illness; 2 developing inner conviction; 3 refraining from making comparisons; 4 prioritizing what is important; 5 sharing stories with others; 6 awareness of shifting one's self-identity; 7 being in tune with the process of learning The concept of readiness to change regarded as fundamental to the link between the learning that arises from living with a chronic illness and 'moving on'. Health professionals described as being in a strong position to facilitate this learning

(Continued)

Table 6.1   *(Cont'd)*

Study details	Summary and comments
5 Persson and Ryden (2006) 'Re-evaluation of life'. Qualitative interview grounded theory study with 26 people with various acquired disabilities	Effective coping involved: (1) self-trust, (2) problem-reducing actions, (3) change of values, (4) social trust, (5) minimization The five categories formed two distinct constructs: acknowledgement of reality versus creation of hope; and trust in oneself versus trust in others. Indicates that a re-evaluation of one's life is to determine what is truly important to achieve or 'an existential shift in life values' (p. 357). Concluded that effective coping 'is more a matter of changing oneself than changing the situation' (p. 358)
6 Rochette et al. (2006) 'Changing perceptions'. Qualitative interview study, using content analysis, involving ten stroke survivors	Seven 'appraisal themes' and five 'coping' themes: 1 appraisal themes were: unpredictability, overwhelming, feeling out of control, threat, turning point, acceptance/resignation, future prospects; 2 coping themes were: active and passive compensation, escape, change how the situation is perceived, utilization of resources In line with transformation and positive reappraisal concepts it was found that the most effective coping strategy for stroke survivors, who cannot resume their pre-stroke lifestyle, was to change how they perceive their situation
7 DeSanto-Madeya (2006) 'The meaning of living with spinal cord injury'. Qualitative phenomenological study of 20 individuals, 5–10 years post spinal cord injury	Seven themes co-existed simultaneously with no discernible difference based on years since injury or level of injury: 1 looking for understanding to a life that is unknown; 2 stumbling along an unlit path; 3 viewing self through a stained glass window; 4 challenging the bonds of love; 5 being chained to the injury; 6 moving forward in a new way of life; 7 reaching a new normalcy
8 Ellis-Hill et al. (2008). 'The Life Thread Model'. This model, grounded in a life narrative approach, used stroke as an example and was based on 10 years of empirical research	Suggests acquired disability be seen as 'a time of transition rather than simply of loss'. Recognizes recovery as a combination of complex physical, psychological and social processes taking place over a long time span. Following stroke, predictability is lost and to move on with life people need to find a 'new me' and learn new rules in an unfamiliar world. Through stories 'individuals create links between their past which is known and their future which is unknown' (p. 153)
9 Kearney (2009) 'Reconfiguring the future'. A PhD thesis based on narrative theory. Model developed from a study with stroke survivors	Extends the work of Ellis-Hill et al. (2008). In this model stroke is portrayed as shattering assumptions about self and life. Post-stroke transitions for stroke survivors and their families involve grief and reconstruction, experienced concurrently. Transition to well-being is depicted as a function of meaning reconstruction and the reconfiguration of new life plots. The valuable role of peer support in the form of 'stroke club' is highlighted in this study

Table 6.1   *(Cont'd)*

Study details	Summary and comments
10 Jeon et al. (2010). 'Renegotiation with self'. A qualitative study of 52 people (and 14 carers) with chronic heart failure or chronic obstructive pulmonary disease	Balancing involved a renegotiation with self about what is normal, and recalibrating personal experiences. For some people many cycles of renegotiation may be required as symptoms worsen
11 Dubouloz et al. (2010). 'Process of transformation model – rehabilitation of chronic illness and disability'. Qualitative meta-synthesis of six studies involving individuals who had experienced either rheumatoid arthritis ($n=25$), myocardial infarction ($n=9$), multiple sclerosis ($n=4$) or spinal cord injury ($n=10$)	This is a specific theory of learning that describes 'the experience of being ill or disabled' (p. 609) as a trigger for transformative change. In particular, the process of change 'is framed by the [person's] critical reflection of bio-psycho-social and spiritual issues encountered in living with the disease or disability' (p. 609). This involves deconstruction and reconstruction of meanings to produce a readiness for change in lifestyle. The outcomes of these reflections are new perspectives, beliefs, feelings and behaviours and a new identity. Readiness for change is an important feature of this model as it is required before the process of changing can begin and transformative outcomes achieved (see also the trans-theoretical model of change, Prochaska et al., 1992)
12 Levack et al. (2010). 'Disconnection and sense of connection with one's body'. Meta-synthesis of 23 qualitative research studies	Eight inter-related themes describe the enduring experience of traumatic brain injury: 1 mind/body disconnect; 2 disconnect with pre-injury identity; 3 social disconnect; 4 emotional sequelae; 5 internal and external resources; 6 reconstruction of identity; 7 reconstruction of a place in the world; 8 reconstruction of personhood Disconnection and reconstruction are central to the experience of traumatic brain injury. Disconnection is experienced within the self in a physical and biographical sense; disconnection from others is experienced spatially, interpersonally and biographically. Reconstruction is the work of recovery; it was a 'daily struggle' because 'reconstruction of personhood required both feeling like a complete individual (*i.e.* reconstructed self-identity) and being accepted as a one by other people (i.e. reconstructed place in the world)' (Levack et al., 2010, p. 996). During these struggles negative emotions were a daily experience

recognizing that spirituality is a difficult concept to describe, Greenstreet (2006) explains that spirituality is 'both covert in constituting the core of the self, and overt, reflected in the way we live, in what we do and how we are with others' (p. 938). As a personal factor, spirituality can allow the person to critically reflect upon their lives and see beyond what Barrow (2008) calls the prevailing cultural narratives of disability.

By now, you might be thinking that research is suggesting that all people experience disability as a positive opportunity to re-invent themselves or as a spiritual awakening. You might also be wondering why your patients are not seeing their circumstances this way. Indeed, although positive transformation may be the case for some, it is not the case for all who experience acquired disability. The stories of three men (Harry, Jamie and David), who sustained spinal cord injuries while playing rugby union (presented by Sparkes and Smith, 2003) illustrates this point well. Pre-injury, rugby defined the lives and the bodies of all three. Post-injury, Harry was living in the future, waiting for the cure that would allow him to resume his pre-injury life. Like Anne (earlier in the chapter), Harry could not see any alternate future self. Jamie felt life had been 'beaten out' out him; he saw his present as empty and lived without ambition for a future (p. 311). David saw life as a journey and disability as a teacher; he talked about himself being reborn and having become a better person. Talking about his post-injury life he said, 'I don't worry about what the future holds…I take each day as it comes, and enjoy the moment' (Sparkes and Smith, 2003, p. 313). So not every person undergoing rehabilitation will go through a transformative process, with Morse (1997) suggesting that the self-reflection required for transformative learning is a later response. This is supported by examination of 'time since diagnosis' for the participants in Dubouloz et al.'s (2010) meta-synthesis about the process of transformation (see Table 6.1). As such, transformative changes associated with more positive outcomes probably come long after discharge from clinical rehabilitation services.

In this section we have looked at the reconstructive and transformational models of change following acquired disability and how they can depict rehabilitation as a journey. These understandings support the belief outlined in Chapter 1 that rehabilitation has a range of meanings, and one such meaning is that rehabilitation is a personal journey. We go on now to consider the work involved in this journey.

6.6 Understanding rehabilitation as 'work' and the role of participation

From the previous section we saw how the personal journey meant that the individual experiencing acquired disability has to work to reduce 'the discrepancy between the person's goal and existing circumstances' (Siegert et al., 2004, p. 1175). However, there is seldom a formal job description and so it is not clear what form this work takes. In a general sense, the work entails the following adaptive tasks: managing symptoms; managing treatment; forming relationships with healthcare providers; managing emotions; maintaining a positive self-image; relating to family members and friends; and preparing for an uncertain future (Moos and Holahan, 2007). In a more specific sense, it may also require sustained physical effort to regain muscle strength and weeks of practice to master a previously taken for granted activity such as holding a cup.

Historically, the work of rehabilitation has been attributed to healthcare professionals who 'rehabilitate' people. Evidence of this is implicit in the early accounts of the rehabilitation literature. Team membership comprised medical, nursing and allied health staff and descriptions of their work reveal that the contributions of patients and their supporters are missing. As explained by Wikman and Faltholm (2006, p. 29), this early model of rehabilitation: 'gives the patient a passive role, where the main concern of the patient is to seek competent help and to adapt himself or herself to the will of the healthcare professionals and co-operate with them in order to get well'.

Traditionally then, rehabilitation has been described as 'the third phase of medicine' (Rusk, 1960). More recently it has been referred to as 'a health strategy' (Stucki et al., 2007, p. 282) and a service. Examples of the aims of such strategies and services include: 'to optimize patient social participation and well-being, and so reduce stress on carer/family' (Wade, 2005, p. 814) and 'to enable people with health conditions experiencing or likely to experience disability achieve and maintain optimal functioning in interaction with the environment' (Stucki et al., 2007, p. 282).

Stories and studies of the lived experience of acquired disability suggest that rehabilitation requires much more than the work of healthcare professionals. In line with O'Connor's (2000, p. 183) thinking that patients 'create their own recovery', Ellis-Hill and colleagues (2008, p. 155) propose rehabilitation is about learning 'how to live a life that is not dominated by their disability'. Here the emphasis is on rehabilitation as a personal journey that entails work. It is also important to recognize the physicality of work done by patients on their rehabilitation journeys (Papadimitriou, 2008), especially when the work is 'highly energetic' (Cameron and Kurlle, 2002, p. 389) and demanding on the body, a body that may also be fatigued and confused by what has happened.

Learning is another major aspect of the work undertaken by patients on their rehabilitation journeys. Problem solving (Wade, 2005) as well as the learning of new skills and strategies (Ward et al., 2009) are required. Initially, the primary purpose of engaging in these activities seems to be the resumption of a pre-injury or illness lifestyle (Doolittle, 1991; Ellis-Hill et al., 2009; Hafsteinsdottir and Grypdonck, 1997; Robison et al., 2009). Hence, rehabilitation is commonly understood to be about 'return' and more specifically the return of physical function. However, as we found in Chapter 1, the 're' in rehabilitation can also mean 'to do again'. This meaning creates opportunities for 'doing' in different ways, for example, doing up buttons using a different technique. Viewed this way, the work of rehabilitation involves the body and the self, with the role of rehabilitation services being to guide and support individuals as they learn different ways. Carlson and colleagues (2006) describe two alternate approaches to the work of learning in rehabilitation: 'learn to participate' and 'participate to learn'. In the first and more dominant model, learning (which happens in controlled environments, commonly a hospital setting) is required before participation in real-life situations. In contrast, the 'participate to learn' approach uses real-life situations as the context for learning. In their review of the literature these authors found that the 'participate to learn' approach was more effective in increasing participation in valued life roles by people with brain injury (Carlson et al., 2006). This suggests that rehabilitation services should be set up in a way that engages patients in everyday activities in their usual context from the earliest possible moment. Carlson et al. (2006) also highlight the importance of support, or the scaffolding as mentioned earlier in the chapter, in this approach. These supports may come from family, friends, carers and colleagues but a very important component is also the person's natural supports, these come from within the person: their own coping abilities, resilience, optimism and hope. Thus, participation in meaningful and productive real-life roles and activities should be the ultimate goal that informs rehabilitation planning as well as providing the context for learning.

We have emphasized this point because meaningful and productive life roles and activities are critical aspects of both the primary goods for life (Siegert et al., 2007) and human well-being (Seligman, 2011) and so they are likely to be crucial ingredients for a person-centred rehabilitation service. We go on to suggest that this 'participate to learn' approach also accommodates the biographical work of rehabilitation as it involves seeing and experiencing the self in different ways in real-life situations. What is less clear is the extent to which rehabilitation services can – or even should – provide these real-life learning opportunities, and this is the topic for the Section 6.7.

6.7   Clinical services guiding and supporting personal rehabilitation journeys

We are now building a picture for rehabilitation being more than a series of intermittent interventions done to patients by health professionals (Pryor, 2005). Rather, rehabilitation is a complex intervention, whereby the interplay of many factors influences how and to what extent a person benefits (Lequerica and Kortte, 2010). Rehabilitation service delivery is an intricate web of processes and subprocesses operating concurrently at both the service and individual patient level. Dobkin and Carmichael (2005) suggest that generally speaking rehabilitation involves restitution, substitution or compensation. Elaborating on this, Ward and colleagues (2009) explain these basic approaches as: reducing activity limitations; acquiring new skills and strategies to lessen the impact of activity limitation; and altering the environment (both physical and social) to reduce the impact of activity limitations on participation in life.

However, regardless of the approach or approaches used, clinical rehabilitation services are, according to the ICF (WHO, 2001), environmental factors that can influence a patient's functioning. This means that all aspects of the built environment, staff, equipment, policies, procedures and practices have the potential to act as facilitators and/or barriers to patient functioning. For example, the terrain outside the rehabilitation ward can determine the extent of independent 'real-life' practice of newly learned skills; the proximity of the gymnasium to the inpatient beds can have an impact upon therapy intensity and frequency; the attitudes of staff regarding the scope of their practice can influence service effectiveness; and rigid visiting hours can have an impact upon time available to interact with family and friends. One of the moves to smooth the patient's journey through the environmental context of healthcare services has been the development of clinical pathways. These focus on providing a route map for health professionals and their administrative staff to follow, enabling best practice guidelines to be implemented and efficiencies to be realized.

An example in rehabilitation is to improve the transition from acute rehabilitation services to community-based rehabilitation and comes from the UK's Stroke Improvement Programme (NHS Improvement, 2011). This initiative includes the implementation of Early Supported Discharge teams; and more recently there is a drive to provide 6-month and then annual reviews for all people recovering from stroke. It will be of some interest to see how well these particular stroke improvement programme initiatives work. Of course, the caveat here is that not everyone 'fits' a pre-determined clinical pathway and a balance has to be struck between this approach and personalized care (see more about this in Section 6.9 of this chapter).

From the perspective that taking the person in their context is crucial to successful modern-day rehabilitation practice, it becomes clear that all the principles we have been discussing for rehabilitation in a healthcare setting also apply to the occupational setting. We have already noted that engagement and achievement are central to human well-being (Seligman, 2011) and for some the return to, or the ability to stay in, paid employment is a vital part of their rehabilitation journey. However, despite the efforts of formal vocational or work rehabilitation programmes and services, there can be many barriers for those wanting to return to work. Shaw and colleagues (2007, p. 66) refer to these barriers as 'the undermining of human potential ... at the system and community level in society'. We suggest greater progress can be made to overcome these barriers if we all strive towards creating more socially inclusive societies. So now we need to consider how the broader sociocultural context can affect rehabilitation services such as social and health inequalities that stem from funding policy, geographical location, or ethnic and cultural differences. We cannot cover all sociocultural contexts in detail in this chapter, instead we offer a few examples that demonstrate a clear impact on rehabilitation patients.

Variation in funding policies can provide us with clear examples of how a person may experience very different rehabilitation services. The UK has a reputation for 'post-code' healthcare, with the extent of service provision often being determined by your address. A recent example of this 'postcode lottery' concerns the provision of physiotherapy services for people with rheumatoid arthritis, a national survey showing that one in three patients have to wait a year or more to see a physiotherapist (National Rheumatoid Arthritis Society and Chartered Society of Physiotherapy, 2011). So a particular geographical location may have more or less healthcare funding resources, depending on the socioeconomic status of the region, to allocate to rehabilitation services. In addition a location may have a long-standing reputation for a particular service, affording greater opportunity of obtaining specialized services versus other locations where there are no specialized staff available. To further illustrate this point we take an example from a stroke user group in the South West of the UK who report no speech and language therapy being available for those with aphasia if you live in the far west of the region; the round trip of more than 4 hours and limited public transport options to where the service can be obtained being a barrier to receiving such a service. This shows how the geographical context, in this case the urban/rural divide, is compounded by the socioeconomic deprivation status of a particular region and the availability of specialist staff.

Similarly, other Western societies also create two tier healthcare, albeit through different types of insurance funding systems. For example, New Zealand has a unique no-fault state Accident Compensation Corporation (ACC) insurance scheme that guarantees rehabilitation to all individuals *who are injured* (www.acc.co.nz n.d.). The ACC system is regarded by many to be a role model for how to resource and provide effective rehabilitation services and yet it results in some interesting variation in the rehabilitation experiences for individuals who live in New Zealand. Those patients who present with very similar functional limitations and rehabilitation needs may end up getting very different levels of services. For example, a person with lower limb amputation due to trauma (such as a motor-cycle accident) is covered by ACC and can get full compensation including up to 80% of pre-injury salary; timely provision of mobility aids and housing modifications, as well as adapted vehicles. In contrast the more poorly resourced Ministry of Health funded system for those with lower limb amputation due to disease, such as diabetes, does not cover salary compensation, may mean access ramps arrive long after they are needed, will only modify houses once, and is unlikely to provide adapted vehicles (Hudson et al., 2008). This situation is further compounded for the Maori and Pacific Islander population of New Zealand. These cultural groups not only have a higher incidence of diabetes-related amputation but also experience health inequalities more generally; and these inequalities are not attributed just to differences in socioeconomic status (Bhopal, 2006; Reid et al., 2000).

Having considered the broader scene we return to our argument that, to be successful, a rehabilitation service must address what matters to the person. An essential starting point is the re-establishment of a 'person's sense of control over his or her body and life' (Ozer, 1999, p. 43). With each patient on their own unique journey, enabling patients to stay connected with their past as they construct their future is paramount in person-centred rehabilitation. However, our understanding of person-centredness within the context of rehabilitation service delivery is far from mature. Person-centred service delivery requires more than individual healthcare professionals or disciplines understanding each patient as a unique person and responding flexibly to their individual needs and preferences. It requires 'whole of service' and system-level approaches to the co-production of person-centred services. With no agreed indicators, the big issues that still need to be addressed concern what would constitute person-centredness in a rehabilitation service and how this might be achieved.

Furthermore, it is unlikely that 'one size will fit all' and so potentially it may be very difficult to get a service to adopt a person-centred model that suits all patients.

Examination of the conceptual and historical perspectives of person-centredness led Leplege et al. (2007) to conclude that 'no consensus can be found either on its meaning or on its implications for rehabilitation' (p. 1564) and thus provides no assistance to help us answer these questions. Various studies (see Table 6.2 for some examples) involving rehabilitation patients, however, may hold some clues for a way forward. Table 6.2 includes studies of the early post-discharge period because a major

Table 6.2 Delivering person-centred services: a selection of examples from the rehabilitation literature.

Study details	Summary and comments
1 Cott (2004) Qualitative study using focus groups, 33 rehabilitation clients with various conditions: spinal cord injury, $n=3$; acquired brain injury, $n=4$; chronic obstructive pulmonary disease, $n=5$; stroke, $n=7$; and arthritis and/or joint replacements, $n=14$	Seven client-centred rehabilitation characteristics as follows: 1 'individualisation of programmes to the needs of each client in order to prepare them for life in the real world; 2 mutual participation with health professionals in decision-making and goal-setting; 3 outcomes that are meaningful to the client; 4 sharing of information and education that is appropriate, timely and according to the client's wishes; 5 emotional support; 6 family and peer involvement throughout the rehabilitation process; and 7 coordination and continuity across the multiple service sectors' (pp. 1418–1419)
2 Hammell (2007) Qualitative meta-synthesis of eight papers (seven studies) involving rehabilitation patients with spinal cord injury	Four important dimensions of rehabilitation from the patient's perspective as follows: 1 specific staff attributes, notably those that made patients feel they were unique people, were highly valued by patients; 2 similarly peers, with spinal cord injury with whom they could identify and who served as role models, were important; 3 they did not, however, like rehabilitation settings that resembled institutions or that used standardized rehabilitation programmes, especially those that lacked relevance, e.g. that discouraged emotional expression or were inadequate in addressing sexual needs; 4 patients wanted programmes that prepared them for life in the real world outside of hospital. In particular, they valued support to envision future life possibilities and to reconnect their past to the future
3 Rittman et al. (2007) Qualitative interview study with 125 stroke survivors	Three major challenges identified 1 month after discharge were: 1 disruption in the construction of self; 2 isolation from others; 3 difficulty accessing activities outside the home
4 Sigurgeirsdottir and Halldorsdottir (2008) Qualitative phenomenological interview study with 12 rehabilitation patients	Rehabilitation patients emphasized the importance of support for their biographical work. In order to be able to cope and adapt to a new life and self, patients expressed a need for: 1 individualized caring; 2 emotional support; 3 a sense of security; 4 progressive care based on realistic and achievable goals

(Continued)

Table 6.2   *(Cont'd)*

Study details	Summary and comments
5 Wain et al. (2008) Qualitative study using interpretative phenomenological analysis with eight patients who had undergone neurological rehabilitation.	Three key attributes of person-centredness as follows: 1 'staff instilling feelings of control and a sense of respect in patients'; and 2 aspects of the 'organisation of the [inpatient] unit, which facilitated a holistic and individual approach to rehabilitation' (p. 1370); 3 in particular, patients drew strength from relationships with other patients. Sharing stories was an important aspect of these relationships
6 Ellis-Hill et al. (2009) Qualitative interview study with 20 people and 13 carers within 1 month of being discharged from hospital following stroke.	Three good and three not so good experiences of transition from hospital to home were reported: 'Discharge was successful if: 1 the sense of momentum was maintained; 2 they felt supported; and 3 they felt informed about what was happening Discharge was seen as seen as difficult when: 1 momentum was perceived to be lost; 2 people did not feel supported; or 3 they felt in the dark about the plans or their recovery' (p. 61)

focus of rehabilitation is preparation for life outside hospital, and this can also help us to understand how best to deliver person-centred services.

Although Table 6.2 is not an exhaustive list of the literature in this area, these studies do convey the importance of capturing the 'stories' that patients can tell us about their experiences of rehabilitation services. It is clear that individuals make their own assessment about whether a rehabilitation service is satisfactory in meeting their needs. There are some common themes about what constitutes 'satisfaction' but the specific details may remain unclear, after all satisfaction is subjective in nature and so inherently an individual experience. Clinicians, who wish to have a better understanding of what this individual experience might be, and how patients assess their satisfaction with services, can do so through building relationships with patients and their families, and it is to the family context that we now turn our attention.

6.8   Placing the person in their family context and involving families in rehabilitation

There is only a small amount of research published in the clinical rehabilitation literature about family-centred approaches to rehabilitation practice for clinicians, so much has to be borrowed from family therapy practice and then applied in principle to the type of rehabilitation we are discussing in this book. However, we want to make an explicit distinction between involving families in rehabilitation and doing family therapy, the latter requires specialist training and is not something we can cover in this book. We acknowledge two family therapists, Ginny Hickman and Bennett Friedmann, for the work they have done in drawing together some of the following material for rehabilitation professionals who want to learn more about family-centred approaches.

The main principle is to think of families as systems and that by understanding this system and how the person and their family members work in this system it is possible to assist the person through their rehabilitation journey (Chenail et al., 1992). Family therapists strive for the individual to always be considered in the context of their family system regardless of where they are in the rehabilitation process. So although medical care might be prioritized at the time of acute hospital admission and it may not be possible to work with the family, there is still an argument for considering the family context as this provides the basis for understanding the patient as a person. For example, as the person moves through their rehabilitation journey so the family functioning changes. Clark and Smith (1999) describe the irrevocable change in family functioning that follows the sudden occurrence of disability (stroke) in a person who was previously a healthy member of the family, and how the care of this person becomes largely the responsibility of the family as the person moves from acute to long-term chronic illness.

Early models of family therapy practice have been criticized for allowing a power imbalance to arise, with health professionals in the dominant position and 'doing' therapy to the family. More recently the 'strengths and solution focused approach' (Munford and Sanders, 1999) and narrative models (White and Epston, 1990) of family therapy, have shown that it is possible to emphasize empowerment, sharing of information and working in partnership with the person in the context of their family. However, it is clear that many health professionals do not feel adequately skilled to work with families, and reports of dissatisfaction with services from families suggest that this is indeed true (Becker and Silburn, 1999). So although this book cannot provide you with training in family therapy for rehabilitation, the following points may help when working with patients in the context of their family:

- interconnections occur between all individuals within a family;
- anything that has an impact on one family member will affect all family members;
- one family member with an illness or injury will have an impact on all family members;
- when someone in a family becomes ill or injured all boundaries, roles, power dynamics, relationships and communication patterns are likely to change;
- talking about what has, and is happening, with everyone will help open lines of communication;
- if possible, attempts should be made to meet and get to know the family, and include them in the rehabilitation plan;
- recognize that the family can play a pivotal role in assisting or obstructing a person's rehabilitation.

(adapted from Hickman and Friedmann, 2010)

These approaches complement the ICF framework, since by thinking about the person in terms of participation (and not impairment or disability) it is then natural to also consider their family and immediate social context.

What these sections and research studies tell us is that rehabilitation services need to support the existential struggle of rehabilitation patients (Sigurgeirsdottir and Halldorsdottir, 2008) as they do the physical, psychological and biographical work of rehabilitation. Furthermore, services must do this in a way that prepares the person for life outside hospital. This can start with fostering a 'can do' attitude and enabling the person to regain control of their present and their future. To this end Ellis-Hill et al. (2008, p. 15) recommend 'endorsing a positive self view'. MacLeod and McPherson (2007) argue that 'a compassionate perspective' is required to guide truly person-centred care that is both empathetic and collaborative. This requires 'something deep' from within rehabilitation staff and needs to 'be expressed as moral action' (MacLeod and McPherson, 2007, p. 1591). Some ideas for operationalizing this moral action in the context of person-centred rehabilitation processes and practices are given in the next section.

6.9   Ideas for making clinical rehabilitation processes and practices person-centred

In this section we move away from the theory and instead offer some ideas for how to be person-centred in your rehabilitation practice. As noted earlier in this chapter, rehabilitation is an intricate web of processes and sub-processes, each with its own potential to be more or less person-centred. However, when rehabilitation is viewed as a collective effort, involving staff, patients and patients' supporters in co-production, the potential of person-centredness can be realized. Rehabilitation practices can then move beyond what Willis and colleagues (2008, p. 94) refer to as 'the rhetoric about patients and families as "partners in care"'.

Thinking of rehabilitation as the co-production of work requires understanding of all the 'ingredients' of that work. The first ingredient is you; you the person who is the health worker *and* you as the health worker. The second is the person who is the patient. The third is the rehabilitation team, ward or service. The fourth is the organization, and the fifth is the policy and funding framework for service provision. It might seem surprising that we have put the health professional as the first ingredient. However, because staff are the face of service, organization and policy, this section starts with the staff. A second reason for starting with the staff is that each of us is responsible for our personal contribution to patient rehabilitation and so it is within our power to control and adapt our practice (and may be one of the reasons you are reading this book).

Idea 1: Get to know yourself

Consider now who are you and what makes you a person, unique from others. We suggest that you, as a person, are a composite of your biology and life experiences and the sense that you make of that. This is what you bring to interactions with rehabilitation patients.

Leaving aside that the ICF is limited in its ability to portray the dynamic nature of your personhood, look at the diagrammatic representation of ICF (WHO, 2001) and use it to think about yourself (see Chapter 2). Think about aspects of your bodily structures and functions: your height, the shape of your feet, how well you see or hear, the strength of your upper arm. Now think about activities and participation in relation to your body, starting with mobility: think about grasping, manipulating, pushing and pulling objects; do you experience any difficulty maintaining a squatting position or walking around an obstacle? Next think about communication and relating to others: initiating, sustaining and ending a conversation or discussion with one or more people, and using various communication machines and technical equipment; do you use similar body language when communicating with strangers, siblings and peers?

Now spend some time thinking about the physical, social and attitudinal aspects of the environments in which you live: consider the products and technology that you use every day, once a week or less often; think about how the attitudes of others have an impact on you; what public policies you agree and disagree with. Finally, think about yourself in terms of personal factors, for example: your methods for coping with taxing situations; your attitudes, values and beliefs about people with disabilities; the role of family and friends in rehabilitation; the role of government in providing for the less able members of a society. Consider now the attitudes, values and beliefs that your socialization as a healthcare professional has instilled in you; whether you bring 'a compassionate perspective' to your work; whether you have been 'trained' to think in a biomedical scientific, reductionist way.

Idea 2: Authentically seek to understand the person who is the patient within the context of their life story

Patients bring their personhood, as well as their impairments and activity limitations to the co-production of work with staff. Like the staff, each patient brings the composite of their biology and life experiences and the sense they make of it. Each also brings their life story and just like staff, patients bring assets and liabilities, enablers and barriers, to rehabilitation. Most importantly, the determination of what is an enabler and what is a barrier is an intrapersonal process, so patients and staff may hold different interpretations. For example, staff may consider 20 cats an environmental hazard for a new wheelchair use; the patient however, may consider the cats as family, providing her with companionship and meaning. This may seem like an extreme example, but we can assure you that many community-based professionals will have encountered similar (i.e. pet related) 'home contexts' and will have been faced with the dilemma arising from interpretation of risk being different between themselves and their patient. In keeping with the theme of this chapter it is beholden to the health professional that they show a commitment to seeking a shared understanding with their patient, and this can be achieved through the assessment process.

As we saw in Chapter 4, assessment is the process healthcare professionals use to get to know their patients, and it is an opportunity to get a sense of the person who is the patient, their life before their current accident or illness as well as their hopes, dreams and plans for the future. Although assessment forms can provide a starting point, they often fall short in capturing a patient's life story. It is all too easy for the time-pressed health professional to just ask closed questions or listen selectively, because they have to fill boxes on an assessment form. The whole assessment process is fraught with even more difficulty when we recognize that the life story of the newly disabled person may be changing, as the person transitions from their old self to their new self. Furthermore, for some rehabilitation patients, life, as they are currently experiencing it, can be foreign and make little sense. This reveals an additional layer of complexity to understanding the person who is currently the patient: their life story, their 'context', may currently be in a state of chaos.

Let us consider *Idea 2* again, how do we 'authentically' seek to understand the person who is the patient within the context of their life story? The answer is simply to listen. Invite patients to share their life stories and listen. Do not interrupt to ask questions on an assessment form. Listen for the meaning that the person attributes to their situation and its causes; listen for evidence of significant people (including pets) and life roles; listen for indicators of environmental enablers and barriers; and listen for the person's strengths and attributes. Listen more than once, listen over and over as patients share their life stories. Listening authentically is the foundation stone of effective rehabilitation practice.

In addition to this 'active' listening role, consider changing the way you prompt the person to tell you more. Traditional clinical assessment questions and prompts are designed to help the clinician in their clinical reasoning process, to drill down to the cause of the problem (to make a diagnosis or classification), to identify a clinical priority, to determine the treatment that best matches the condition. These questions tend to be worded as 'closed questions', inviting a 'yes' or 'no' answer, such as the patient with low back pain who has to tell the physiotherapist where they feel the 'worst' pain (and so discounting all the other pains or symptoms that may matter to them). Asking the patient 'please will you tell me about your back pain?' is an open-ended question, an invitation to talk freely about their low back pain experience. These types of questions are typical of qualitative approaches to health research enquiry, whereby the researcher endeavours to maintain a mutual power balance in their relationship with the research participant. Trying this approach as a clinician is initially hard work, the assessment schedule can be disrupted and even not completed (from the clinician's traditional point of view). Yet, so much more can be learnt about what matters to that patient when you ask open-ended questions, such as 'what do you expect from rehabilitation?' as some patients may not even know why they have been referred to a particular service, such as physiotherapy. This question may also reveal the patient's beliefs about their condition and how they make sense of a proposed treatment (for more on this see Weinman et al, 1996). In the example of the patient with low back pain, if they thought their back was 'worn out' because the doctor had told them it was showing signs of 'wear and tear' due to the degenerative changes of old age, then they might also think that the physiotherapist's exercises would 'wear' their backs out even further. In this situation it is unlikely to make sense for the patient to engage in exercise-based rehabilitation.

Idea 3: Take responsibility for building a trusting relationship that enables patients to do the physical and biographical work of rehabilitation

The next step, after authentically seeking to understand the person who is the patient within the context of their life story, is to help that person to build the scaffolding that enables them to do the physical and biographical work of rehabilitation. Part of this means we have to take responsibility for building a trusting relationship that enables patients to do that work.

This starts with taking individual responsibility for being genuinely trustworthy and demonstrating this to patients. To do this, we need a wide repertoire of interpersonal skills for connecting with people. In *Idea 1* we asked you to consider your own interpersonal skills, this type of self-assessment can help you to uncover any biases or unhelpful attitudes, values or belief that may make patients wary of engaging with you or trusting you. Listening authentically is an important skill for building trusting relationships with patients. Displaying genuine concerns for others may help a patient to view you as trustworthy. Developing a different approach to your clinical encounters and consultation techniques is worth considering. In the literature that explores the reasons why patients do not adhere to their treatment it is clear that the therapeutic alliance, or 'concordance' between patient and health professional, is crucial for establishing the rapport that promotes treatment adherence (Myers and Midence, 1998). This means mutual decision making, allowing the patient to play an active role in his or her rehabilitation and to be empowered to engage in their rehabilitation.

Idea 4: Consider ways of incorporating into your practice strategies that empower, or 'activate' patients

Activation or empowerment (Michie et al., 2003) can be achieved by stimulating patients to make their own plans for managing their condition and for promoting their self-efficacy (Bandura, 1997). The idea here is that they can then implement their plans and be motivated and confident about their ability to carry them out (Michie et al., 2003) and more discussion about motivational approaches for promoting self-efficacy can be found in Chapter 4.

Idea 5: Acknowledge, value, respect and support the biographical as well as the physical and psychological work of rehabilitation

Acknowledging, valuing, respecting and supporting the biographical as well as the psychological and physical work of rehabilitation is a relatively new paradigm for rehabilitation service delivery. It demands more than the traditional strong points of rehabilitation service delivery, namely ameliorating bodily impairments, activity limitations and disabling physical environments. The new paradigm does not mean diluting traditional strengths, it means adding to them. We are not advocating 'throwing the baby out with the bathwater' as many established biomedical approaches are still needed. What we do mean is seeing the person who is the patient as more than primarily a dysfunctional body; it means supporting them to make sense of their whole situation, to develop a sense of coherence, to experience a sense of wholeness, to link yesterday with today and tomorrow. It also means putting the patient in the centre of rehabilitation practice, taking account of this person in their context and that this is acknowledged, valued, respected and supported in every structure, process and sub-process of service delivery. Some attempts have been made to do this in health-care more generally in the UK and the following provide four examples.

The first is the Expert Patients' Programme that is a self-management programme for people living with chronic conditions. It aims to increase patient confidence, improve their QoL and help them to manage their condition more effectively (NHS Choices, 2011). Although this has dramatically improved patient satisfaction with services, it is not yet clear if it has demonstrated meaningful benefits in terms of health outcomes for these patients. However, an internal evaluation of the programme indicates general practitioner consultations have been reduced by 7%, physiotherapy use by 9%, outpatient visits by 10% and 16% fewer emergency hospital attendances (Department of Health, 2010).

Second, there has been a proliferation of patient-reported outcome measures (PROMs), and these have been covered in more detail in Chapter 5. However, the point to be made in this chapter is that PROMs enable patients to evaluate the benefit of receiving healthcare in a way that is meaningful to them. Many of these measures were developed using qualitative research methods, so take account of experiences of patients who have similar conditions, and these measures are being used for clinical services as well as for health services research.

Our third example is the more recent move for patient and public involvement (PPI) in applied health research and care. INVOLVE (www.invo.org.uk) and the James Lind Alliance (www.lindalliance.org) are two UK-based organizations that are worth taking a look at if you are considering undertaking any rehabilitation-related research and want to engage service users at an early stage of the research planning. As an example of the philosophy underpinning the PPI movement, Gibson (2011) gives the following explanation.

> Involving people in health and social care research is about giving the people who are meant to benefit from this research a say in shaping the research agenda. It requires lay people to be involved on an equal basis to academics and health care professionals. This includes not just participating in research that has been initiated by academics but also in shifting the power balance so that users and carers can initiate research and work collaboratively with academics. The interaction between researchers and the public should be based on one of mutual benefit rather than researchers simply extracting useful knowledge to their own advantage. This view is partly based on an ethical principle that the public has a right to influence research priorities. It also depends on the idea that

ensuring that research addresses patients' needs and perceptions increases the effective use of research evidence in practice. Delivering this requires developing effective user involvement in all stages of the research process. (Reproduced from the Peninsula Collaboration for Leadership in Applied Health Research and Care (PenCLAHRC) website with permission from Andy Gibson, 2011)

In other words, if we expect patients to engage and adhere to their rehabilitation intervention then it makes sense that patients are involved from an early point in contributing to the development of that intervention or rehabilitation service.

Our fourth example concerns the strong drive towards personalized care, also known as the 'personalization agenda'. The UK's Care Quality Commission describes this as care that meets individualized needs and that 'we want health care and social care to be more person-centred. Care should be based on each person's unique needs, rather than a "one-size fits all" approach' (Care Quality Commission, n.d.). One way this is being implemented is through 'personal health care budgets'. These allow patients to choose what services, including rehabilitation services, they wish to spend their allocation of health and social care money on. There is a clear expectation that patients should be offered a choice and the NHS Future Forum has recommended, subject to evidence from pilot projects, that there will be 'a priority to extend personal health budgets, including integrated budgets across health and social care' (Department of Health, 2011).

This personalized care agenda promises a move away from institutionalized care practices, but it remains to be seen whether this can be achieved or what impact the agenda will have on 'patient-centred' rehabilitation. The interested reader may wish to follow up on how these social care policies might affect rehabilitation services, for example the special issue of the *Journal of Care Services Management* examines the 'personalized' future (Johnson, 2010) and a Dartington review considers the future of UK adult social care up to 2020 (Humphries, 2010). Similarly, Cornes (2011) discusses the challenges of managing the change that is required for personalization, recounting a sad but 'true story of hospital discharge' when nobody told relatives anything. Cornes goes on to discuss how a health and social care cultural transformation might be achieved for delivering the personalization agenda, with specific mention of the importance of issues we covered in Chapter 3: interprofessional working and establishing communities of practice (Cornes, 2011).

6.10   Can we do person-centred rehabilitation?

We end the 'person in context' theme by concluding that there is a strong case that we *should* be doing person-centred rehabilitation, yet the questions remain unanswered as to whether we can do this, or indeed want to do this. The challenge for rehabilitation professionals in the future will be to answer these questions. However, it is clear that the shift towards patient autonomy and empowerment is likely to stay with us. The roll out of personal health care budgets in the UK places a considerable degree of the purchasing power for choosing rehabilitation services in the patient's hands, the recognition of carers and families, and the drive towards integration of support services across sectors (health, social care and education), all point towards the need for interprofessional rehabilitation that puts the person who is the patient at the centre of rehabilitation policy, service delivery and practice.

Additional resources

Ramsden, E. (1999). *The Person as Patient: Psychosocial Perspectives for the Health Care Professional*. London: WB Saunders Company.

INVOLVE: www.invo.org.uk (accessed 29 February 2012).

James Lind Alliance: www.lindalliance.org (accessed 29 February 2012).*The International Journal of Person Centred Medicine.*

References

Accident Compensation Corporation (n.d.) http://www.acc.co.nz/about-acc/overview-of-acc/introduction-to-acc/index.htm (accessed 23 May 2012).

Bandura, A. (1997). *Self-efficacy: The Exercise of Control*. New York: W. H. Freeman.

Barrow, R. (2008). Listening to the voice of living with aphasia: Anne's story. *International Journal of Language and Communication Disorders*, *43*(S1), 30–46.

Becker, S. and Silburn, R. (1999) *We're in this Together*. London: Carer's National Association.

Bensing, J. M., Verhaak, P. F. M., van Dulman A. M. and Visser, A. P. (2000). Communication: the royal pathway to patient-centred medicine. *Patient Education and Counseling*, *39*, 1–3.

Bhopal, R. (2006). Racism, socioeconomic deprivation, and health in New Zealand. *The Lancet*, *367*, 1958–1959.

Cameron, I. D. (2010). Models of rehabilitation – commonalities of interventions that work and of those that do not. *Disability and Rehabilitation*, *32*(12), 1051–1058.

Cameron, I. D. and Kurlle, S. E. (2002). Rehabilitation and older people. *Medical Journal of Australia*, *177*(7), 461–466.

Care Quality Commission (n.d.). *Person-Centred Care*. Newcastle Upon Tyne: Care Quality Commission. http://archive.cqc.org.uk/stateofcare/carethatmeetsanindividualsneeds.cfm (accessed 10 March 2012).

Carlson, P. M., Boudreau, M. L., Davis, J., Johnston, J., Lemsky, C., McColl, M. A., Minnes, P. and Smith, C. (2006). 'Participate to learn': a promising practice for community ABI rehabilitation. *Brain Injury*, *20*(11), 1111–1117.

Chenail, R. J., Levinson, K. and Muchnick, R. (1992). Family systems rehabilitation. *The American Journal of Family Therapy*, *20*(2), 157–167.

Clark, M. and Smith, D.S. (1999). Changes in family functioning for stroke rehabilitation patients and their families. *International Journal of Rehabilitation Research*, *22*, 171–179.

Clarke, D. (2010). Achieving teamwork in stroke units: the contribution of opportunistic dialogue. *Journal of Interprofessional Care*, *24*(3), 285–297.

Cornes, M. (2011). The challenge of managing change: what can we do differently to ensure personalisation? *Journal of Integrated Care*, *19*(2), 22–29.

Cott, C. A. (2004). Client-centred rehabilitation: client perspectives. *Disability and Rehabilitation*, *26*(24), 1411–1422.

D'Alisa, S., Baudo, S., Mauro, A. and Miscio, G. (2005). How does stroke restrict participation in long-term post-stroke survivors? *Acta Neurologica Scandinavia*, *112*, 157–162.

DeJong, G., Horn, S. D., Gassaway, J. A., Slavin M. D. and Dijkers, M. P. (2004). Towards a taxonomy of rehabilitation interventions: using an inductive approach to examine the "black box" of rehabilitation. *Archives of Physical Medicine and Rehabilitation*, *85*, 678–686.

Department of Health. (2004). *NHS Physiotherapy Services. Summary Information for 2003–04, England*. London: Department of Health.

Department of Health. (2010). *Evaluation of the Expert Patients Programme*. London: Department of Health. http://webarchive.nationalarchives.gov.uk/+/www.dh.gov.uk/en/Aboutus/MinistersandDepartmentLeaders/ChiefMedicalOfficer/Archive/ProgressOnPolicy/ProgressBrowsableDocument/DH_5380885 (accessed 1 July 2011).

Department of Health. (2008). http://webarchive.nationalarchives.gov.uk/+/www.dh.gov.uk/en/SocialCare/Socialcarereform/Personalisation/DH_080573 (accessed 23 May 2012).

DeSanto-Madeya, S. (2006). The meaning of living with spinal cord injury 5 to 10 years after injury. *Western Journal of Nursing Research*, *28*(3), 265–289.

Dictionary.com. Person. (n.d.). Oakland, CA: Lexico Publishing Group. http://dictionary.reference.com/browse/person (accessed 5 March 2012).

Dictionary.com. Personhood. (n.d.). Oakland, CA: Lexico Publishing Group. http://dictionary.reference.com/browse/personhood (accessed 5 March 2012).

Dictionary.com. Oakland, CA: Lexico Publishing Group. http://dictionary. reference.com/browse/person (accessed 5 March 2012).

Dobkin, B. and Carmichael, T. (2005). Principles of recovery after stroke. In: M. Barnes, B. Dobkin and J. Bogousslavsky (Editors). *Recovery after Stroke*. Cambridge: Cambridge University Press, pp. 47–49.

Doolittle, N. (1991). The experience of recovery following lacunar stroke: Implications for acute care. *Journal of Neuroscience*, *23*(4), 235–240.

Dubouloz, C-J., King, J., Ashe, B., Paterson, B., Chevier, J. and Moldoveanu, M. (2010). The process of transformation in rehabilitation: what does it look like? *International Journal of Therapy and Rehabilitation*, *17*(11), 604–613.

Duggan, C. H., Albright, K. J. and Lequerica, A. (2008). Using the ICF to code and analyse women's disability narratives. *Disability and Rehabilitation*, *30*(12), 978–990.

Ellis-Hill, C., Payne, S. and Ward, C. (2008). Using stroke to explore the Life Thread Model: an alternative approach to understanding rehabilitation following an acquired disability. *Disability and Rehabilitation*, *30*(2), 150–159.

Ellis-Hill, C., Robson, J., Wiles, R., McPherson, K., Hyndman, D. and Ashburn, A. on behalf of the Stroke Association Rehabilitation Research Centre Team. (2009). Going home to get on with life: patients and carers experiences of being discharged from hospital following stroke. *Disability and Rehabilitation*, *31*(2), 61–72.

Faircloth, C. A., Boystein, C., Rittman, M., Young, M. E. and Gubrium, J. (2004). Sudden illness and biographical flow in narratives of stroke recovery. *Sociology of Health and Illness*, *26*(2), 242–261.

Faull, K. and Hills, M. D. (2006). The role of the spiritual dimension of the self as the prime determinant of health. *Disability and Rehabilitation*, *28*(11), 729–740.

Folkman, S. and Moskowitz, J. T. (2000). Positive affect and the other side of coping. *American Psychologist*, *55*(6), 647–654.

The Free Dictionary. Personhood (n.d.) Huntington Valley, PA: Farlex. http://www.thefree dictionary.com/personhood (accessed 51 March 2012).

The Free Dictionary. Huntington Valley, PA: Farlex. http://www.thefreedictionary.com/ personhood (accessed 5 March 2012).

Gibson, A. (2011). *Patient and Public Involvement in Research*. Exeter: PenCLAHRC. http://clahrc-peninsula.nihr.ac.uk/patient-public-involvment-in-research.php (accessed 28 September 2011).

Greenstreet, W. (2006). From spirituality to coping strategy: making sense of chronic illness. *British Journal of Nursing*, *15*(17), 938–942.

Guidetti, S., Asaba, E. and Tham, K. (2009). Meaning of context in recapturing self-care after stroke or spinal cord injury. *The American Journal of Occupational Therapy*, *61*, 323–332.

Hafsteinsdottir, T. B. and Grypdonck, M. (1997). Being a stroke patient: a review of the literature. *Journal of Advanced Nursing*, *26*, 580–588.

Hammell, K. W. (2007). Experience of rehabilitation following spinal cord injury: a meta-synthesis of qualitative findings. *Spinal Cord*, *45*, 260–274.

Hasler, R. M., Exadaktylos, A. K., Bouamra, O., Benneker, L. M., Clancy, M., Sieber, R., Zimmermann, H. and Lecky, F. (2011). Epidemiology and predictors of spinal injury in adult major trauma patients: European cohort study. *European Journal of Spine*, *20*(12), 2174–2180.

Hickman, G. and Friedmann, B. (2010). *Family Systems and Rehabilitation. Module Coursebook REHX709*. Christchurch: Rehabilitation Teaching and Research Unit, University of Otago.

Hudson, S., Dean, S., Dew, K., Montgomery, H. and Howden-Chapman, P. (2008). 'I can't sort of do want I wanted to do …' housing needs and experiences of people with disability in New Zealand: a qualitative study following lower limb amputation. *Warwick 5th Healthy Housing Conference*. Presentation, Warwick University, March 2008.

Humphries, R. (2010). *Dartington Review on the Future of Adult Social Care: Overview Report. Research in Practice for Adults*. Devon: The Dartington Hall Trust.

Jeon, Y-H., Jowsey, T., Yen, L., Glasgow, N. J., Essue, B., Kljakovic, M., Pearce-Brown, C., Mirzaei, M., Usherwood, T. Jan, S., Kraus, S. G. and Aspin, C. (2010). Achieving a balanced life in the face of chronic illness. *Australian Journal of Public Health*, *16*, 66–74.

Johnson, N. (2010). Personalisation special issue. *Journal of Care Services Management*, *4*(3), 197–198.

Kearney, P. M. (2009). *Reconfiguring the Future: Stories of Post-Stroke Transition* (PhD thesis). Adelaide: University of South Australia.

Kirschner, K. (1997). Musing on personhood. *Topics in Stroke Rehabilitation*, *4*(2), 92–93.

Kralik, D., Telford, K., Campling, F., Koch, T., Price, K. and Crouch, P. (2005). 'Moving on': the transition to living well with chronic illness. *The Australian Journal of Holistic Nursing*, *12*(2), 13–22.

Lauver, D. R., Ward, S. E., Heidrich, S. M., Keller, M. L., Bowers, B. J., Flatley Brennan, P., Kirchhoff, K. T. and Wells, T. J. (2002). Patient-centred interventions. *Research in Nursing and Health*, *25*, 246–255.

Lazarus, R.S., and Folkman, S. (1984). *Stress, Appraisal, and Coping*. New York: Springer.

Leidy, N. K. and Haase, J. E. (1999). Functional status from the patient's perspective: the challenge of preserving personal integrity. *Research in Nursing and Health*, *22*, 67–77.

Leplege, A., Gzil, F., Cammelli, M., Lefeve, C., Pachoud, B. and Ville, I. (2007). Person-centredness: conceptual and historical perspectives. *Disability and Rehabilitation*, *29* (20–21), 1555–1565.

Lequerica, A. H. and Kortte, K. (2010). Therapeutic engagement: a proposed model of engagement in medical rehabilitation. *American Journal of Physical Medicine and Rehabilitation*, *89*, 415–422.

Levack, W. M. M., Kayes, N. M. and Fadyl, J. K. (2010). Experience of recovery and outcome following traumatic brain injury: a metasynthesis of qualitative research. *Disability and Rehabilitation*, *32*(12), 986–999.

MacLeod, R. and McPherson, K. M. (2007). Care and compassion: part of person-centred rehabilitation, inappropriate response or a forgotten art? *Disability and Rehabilitation*, *29*(20–21), 1589–1595.

Masala, C. and Petretto, D. R. (2008). From disablement to enablement: conceptual models of disability in the 20th century. *Disability and Rehabilitation*, *30*(17), 1233–1244.

McPherson, K. M., Brander, P. Taylor, W. and McNaughton, H. (2004). Consequences of stroke, arthritis and chronic pain – are there important similarities? *Disability and Rehabilitation*, *26*(16), 988–999.

Mead, N. and Bower, P. (2000). Patient-centredness: a conceptual framework and review of the empirical literature. *Social Science and Medicine*, *51*, 1087–1110.

Michie, S., Miles, J. and Weinman, J. (2003). Patient-centredness in chronic illness: what is it and does it matter? *Patient Education and Counselling*, *51*, 197–206.

Moos, R. H. and Holahan, C. J. (2007). Adaptive tasks and methods of coping with illness and disability. In: E. Martz and H. Livneh (Editors). *Coping with Chronic Illness and Disability: Theoretical, Empirical and Clinical Aspects*. New York: Springer, pp. 107–126.

Morse, J. (1997). Responding to threats to integrity of self. *Advances in Nursing Science*, *19*(4), 21–36.

Munford, R. and Sanders, J. (1999) *Supporting Families*. Palmerston North: Dunmore Press.

Myers, L. B. and Midence, K. (1998). Methodological and conceptual issues in adherence. In: L. B. Myers and K. Midence (Editors). *Adherence to Treatment in Medical Conditions*. Amsterdam: Harwood Academic Press.

National Rheumatoid Arthritis Society in collaboration with the Chartered Society of Physiotherapy. (2011). *RA and Physiotherapy: A National Survey*. Maidenhead National Rheumatoid Arthritis Society.

NHS Choices. *The Expert Patients Programme*. London: NHS Choices. www.nhs.uk. (2011). http://www.nhs.uk/Conditions/Expert-patients-programme-/Pages/Introduction.aspx (accessed 1 July 2011).

NHS Improvement. (2011) *NHS Improvement – Stroke. Supporting the Development of Stroke Care Networks*. London: NHS improvement. http://www.improvement.nhs.uk/stroke/ESD/tabid/160/Default.aspx (accessed 5 November 2011).

Norton, L. (2010). *Spinal Cord Injury Australia 2007–08. Injury research and statistics series no. 52. Cat no. INJCAT 128*. Canberra: Australian Institute of Health and Welfare.

O'Connor, S. E. (2000). Mode of care delivery in stroke rehabilitation nursing: a development of Kirkevold's unified theoretical perspective of the role of the nurse. *Clinical Effectiveness in Nursing*, *4*, 180–188.

Ozer, M. N. (1999). Patient participation in the management of stroke rehabilitation. *Topics in Stroke Rehabilitation*, *6*(1), 43–59.

Papadimitriou, C. (2008). 'It was hard but you did it': the co-production of 'work' in a clinical setting among spinal cord injured adults and their physical therapists. *Disability and Rehabilitation*, *30*(5), 365–374.

Patston, P. (2007). Constructive Functional Diversity: a new paradigm beyond disability and impairment. *Disability and Rehabilitation*, *29*(20–21), 1625–1633.

Persson, L-O. and Ryden, A. (2006). Themes of effective coping in physical disability: an interview study of 26 persons who have learnt to live with their disability. *Scandinavian Journal of Caring Science*, *20*, 355–363.

Prochaska, J. O., DiClemente, C. C. and Norcross, J. (1992). In search of how people change. *American Psychologist*, *47*(9), 1102–1114.

Pryor, J. (2005). *A Grounded Theory of Nursing's Contribution to Inpatient Rehabilitation* (PhD thesis). Melbourne: Deakin University.

Pryor, J. (2008). A nursing perspective on the relationship between nursing and allied health in inpatient rehabilitation. *Disability and Rehabilitation*, *30*(4), 314–322.

Reid, P., Robson, B. and Jones, C. P. (2000) Disparities in health: common myths and uncommon truths. *Pacific Health Dialog*, *7*(1), 38–47.

Rittman, M., Boystein, C., Hinojosa, R., Hinojosa, M. S. and Huan, J. (2007). Transition experiences of stroke survivors following discharge home. *Topics in Stroke Rehabilitation*, *14*(2), 21–31.

Robison, J., Wiles, R., Elllis-Hill, C., McPherson, K., Hyndman, D. and Ashburn, A. (2009). Resuming previously valued activities post-stroke: who or what helps? *Disability and Rehabilitation*, *31*(19), 1555–1566.

Rochette, A., St-Cyr-Tribble, D., Desrosiers, J., Bravo, G. and Bourget, A. (2006). Adaptation and coping following a first stroke: a qualitative analysis of a phenomenological orientation. *International Journal of Rehabilitation Research*, *29*, 247–249.

Rusk, H. A. (1960). Rehabilitation: the third phase of medicine. *Rhode Island Medical Journal*, *43*, 385–387.

Schulz, E. K. (2005). The meaning of spirituality for individuals with disabilities. *Disability and Rehabilitation*, *27*(21), 1283–1295.

Seymour, W. (1998). *Remaking the Body: Rehabilitation and Change*. St. Leonards, NSW: Allen and Unwin.

Secrest, J. A. and Thomas, S. P. (1999). Continuity and discontinuity: the quality of life following stroke. *Rehabilitation Nursing*, *24*(6), 240–246.

Seligman, M. (2011). *Flourish*. North Sydney: William Heinemann.

Shaw, L., McWilliam, C., Sumison, T. and MacKinnon, J. (2007). Optimizing environments for consumer participation and self-direction in finding employment. *OTJR: Occupation, Participation and Health*, *27*(2), 59–70.

Siegert, R. J., McPherson, K. M. and Taylor, W. J. (2004). Toward a cognitive-affective model of goal-setting in rehabilitation: is self-regulation theory a key step? *Disability and Rehabilitation*, *26*(20), 1175–1183.

Siegert, R. J., Ward, T., Levack, W. M. and McPherson, K. M. (2007). A good lives model of clinical and community rehabilitation. *Disability and Rehabilitation*, *29*(20–21), 1604–1615.

Siegert, R. J., Ward, T. and Playford, D. (2010). Human rights and rehabilitation outcomes. *Disability and Rehabilitation*, *32*(12), 965–971.

Sigurgeirsdottir, J. and Halldorsdottir, S. (2008). Existential struggle and self-reported needs of patients in rehabilitation. *Journal of Advanced Nursing*, *61*(4), 384–392.

Simmonds, F., Stevermuer, T. and Rankin, N. (2009) *The AROC Annual Report: The State of Rehabilitation in Australia in 2008*. University of Wollongong: Centre for Health Service Development.

Sparkes, A. C. and Smith, B. (2003). Men, sport, spinal cord injury and narrative time. *Qualitative Research*, *3*(3), 295–320.

Souraya, S., Epstein, D. and Miranda, J. (2006). Eliciting patient treatment preferences: a strategy to integrate evidence-based and patient-centred care. *Worldviews on Evidence-Based Nursing*, *3*(3), 116–123.

Stucki, G., Cieza, A. and Melvin, J. (2007). The International Classification of Functioning, Disability and Health: a unifying model for the conceptual description of the rehabilitation strategy. *Journal of Rehabilitation Medicine*, *39*, 279–285.

Wain, H. R., Kneebone, I. I. and Billings, J. (2008). Patient experience of neurological rehabilitation: a qualitative investigation. *Archives of Physical Medicine and Rehabilitation*, *89*, 1366–1371.

Wade, D. (2005). Describing rehabilitation interventions. *Clinical Rehabilitation*, *19*, 811–818.

Wade, D. T., and Halligan, P. (2003). New wine in old bottles: the WHO ICF as an explanatory model of human behaviour. *Clinical Rehabilitation*, *17*, 349–354.

Ward, A. B., Barnes, M. P., Stark, S. C. and Ryan, S. (2009). *Oxford Handbook of Clinical Rehabilitation (2nd edition)*. Oxford: Oxford University Press.

Weinman, J., Petrie, K. J., Moss-Morris, R. and Horne, R. (1996). The illness perception questionnaire: a new method for assessing the cognitive representation of illness. *Psychology and Health*, *11*, 431–445.

White, M. and Epston, D. (1990) *Narrative means to Therapeutic Ends*. Adelaide: Dulwich Centre Publications.

Whyte, J. and Hart, T. (2003). It's more than a black box; it's a Russian doll: defining rehabilitation treatments. *American Journal of Physical Medicine and Rehabilitation*, *82*, 639–652.

Wikman, A. M. and Faltholm, Y. (2006). Patient empowerment in rehabilitation: "Somebody told me to get rehabilitated". *Advances in Physiotherapy*, *8*, 23–32.

Willis, E., Dwyer, J. and Dunn, S. (2008). The collectivity of healthcare: multidisciplinary team care. In: R. Sorensen and R. Iedema (Editors.) *Managing Clinical Processes in Health Services*. Chatswood: Elsevier, pp. 87–104.

World Health Organization. (2001). *International Classification of Functioning, Disability and Health*. Geneva: World Health Organization.

Chapter 7

Conclusion: rethinking rehabilitation

Sarah G. Dean,[1] Richard J. Siegert[2]
and William J. Taylor[3]

[1]*Senior Lecturer in Health Services Research, University of Exeter Medical School,
United Kingdom;* [2]*Professor of Psychology and Rehabilitation, School of Rehabilitation and
Occupation Studies and School of Public Health and Psychosocial Studies, AUT University, Auckland,
New Zealand;* [3]*Associate Professor in Rehabilitation Medicine, Rehabilitation Teaching and
Research Unit, University of Otago Wellington and Consultant Rheumatologist and
Rehabilitation Physician, Hutt Valley District Health Board, Wellington, New Zealand*

7.1 Introduction

This final chapter offers some concluding thoughts about the core themes presented in this book. Each theme will be summarized and some key messages given. We go on to present two case studies that have been 'mapped' onto the International Classification of Functioning, Disability and Health (ICF, World Health Organization (WHO), 2001). In doing this we aim to demonstrate how these core themes in rehabilitation can be brought together to help us in our clinical practice. We will also revisit our earlier discussion about the definition of rehabilitation in the context of current and future healthcare, and go on to consider some of the limitations of this textbook and offer some ideas about the future of interprofessional rehabilitation.

7.2 The ICF as a theoretical framework and language for rehabilitation

In Chapter 2 Will Taylor and Szilvia Geyh described the ICF and explained how it can be used in rehabilitation practice. The ICF is both a model for understanding the manifestations of health conditions in people's lives and also a detailed classification system or taxonomy of the various components within the model. The ICF permits a

Interprofessional Rehabilitation: A Person-Centred Approach, First Edition.
Edited by Sarah G. Dean, Richard J. Siegert and William J. Taylor.
© 2012 John Wiley & Sons, Ltd. Published 2012 by John Wiley & Sons, Ltd.

much clearer understanding of the meaning of 'functioning'. It is clear that pathological changes in physiological structures and body functions (e.g. muscle strength) are not necessary to effect changes at whole body activity level (e.g. moving around the house) or in terms of social participation (e.g. employment). In many ways, this model is the foundation of contemporary rehabilitation practice. The key messages from this chapter are as follows:

- ICF framework of thinking – functioning should be considered at organ, whole body and social levels; functioning is determined by the interaction between health conditions and context (the environment and personal factors) and not solely by health;
- the ICF provides a shared language – this can facilitate teamwork;
- the ICF can be used as an assessment tool – providing a detailed description of a patient's status;
- the ICF concept of functioning is not linear – participation restriction may occur with minimal or no impairment (e.g. fibromyalgia) and vice versa (e.g. spinal cord injury).

7.3   Interprofessional teamwork in rehabilitation

In Chapter 3 Claire Ballinger and Sarah Dean offered some perspectives on what is meant by the interprofessional team and how they work in rehabilitation. They explored issues of professional and disciplinary identity, described some of the roles within teams and the characteristics of good teamwork. The development of interprofessional teamwork in rehabilitation was also described and the debate extended to discuss the importance of collaboration in the contexts of education, practice and research. The key messages arising from this theme are that:

- the whole of the team is greater than the sum of its parts;
- interprofessional teams can generate new knowledge;
- they include the patient, carer and family;
- they require thinking outside of a single professional or disciplinary box;
- they help create communities of practice;
- they do not mean everyone on a team can do everything.

7.4   Processes in rehabilitation: goal setting and its mediators

Key processes in rehabilitation were discussed in Chapter 4 by William Levack, who has specialized in investigating the role and purposes of goal setting as one of the cornerstones of rehabilitation practice, along with Sarah Dean. The chapter also covers some of the mediators, or factors that affect the process of rehabilitation, for example motivation and adherence to treatment. Similarly the chapter discussed other key processes such as assessment and evaluation, including general principles about intervention delivery. The key messages from this theme are:

- rehabilitation is a dynamic process, as depicted by the rehabilitation cycle or spiral;
- the process comprises assessment, goal planning, interventions and evaluation;
- the process requires health professionals to be creative and flexible in their work, and
- to actively engage with patients and their families in the planning and implementation of interventions;
- robust plans for treatment or intervention should be developed, based on the needs and preferences of patients that are also adjustable as goals are met or changed.

7.5 Outcome measurement to evaluate rehabilitation and show it makes a difference

Richard Siegert and Jo Adams examined the use of outcome measures in rehabilitation and some of the important issues arising for clinicians and patients in Chapter 5. In particular, this chapter considered why the use of outcome measures is becoming a routine part of good practice in rehabilitation and also how and who decides which are the important outcomes to measure. The technical aspects of outcome measures, a field known as 'psychometrics', was briefly reviewed with a rehabilitation focus. Lastly, some specific issues, such as the cultural relevance of outcome measures, were highlighted. As with the other chapters in this book the authors recommended the ICF as a useful conceptual framework to guide the application of outcome measures in rehabilitation. The key messages from this core theme include the following:

- there are important ethical, clinical, scientific and financial reasons for using outcome measures routinely;
- outcome measures allow the patient's or client's voice to be heard – and patients/clients must be actively involved in their development;
- rehabilitation outcome measures must be rigorously evaluated according to psychometric standards of reliability, validity, etc;
- the ICF provides a practical framework for defining the target of a rehabilitation intervention and for specifying the level of functioning at which the outcome of that intervention is to be measured;
- the use of outcome measures is no substitute for clinical expertise, reasoning or wisdom.

7.6 The importance of the individual person in their context and how to do person-centred rehabilitation

In Chapter 6 Julie Pryor and Sarah Dean explored what is meant by person-centred. A wide range of terms were discussed although there were limitations in being able to offer clear definitions. The lived experience of acquired disability was considered along with how much might be known about an individual who we work with in rehabilitation. A large portion of the chapter reviewed the notion that rehabilitation is a 'personal journey' of reconstruction and transformation of the self and that there is much work to do along the journey. The role of clinical services in supporting and guiding patients through the work of rehabilitation was discussed and examples given from a number of different contexts, including the family and funding environment. The chapter ended by asking the reader to think about rehabilitation as a co-production of work between the patient and rehabilitation professionals and to focus on some of the strategies a rehabilitation professional might employ to engage with this production. These strategies were: knowing yourself; being authentic; active listening; building trust; empowering and activating patients; acknowledging, valuing and respecting all aspects of the biographical, physical and psychological work of rehabilitation. The key messages from this theme are as follows:

- there is a strong case for doing person-centred rehabilitation that involves:
  - a shift towards patient autonomy and empowerment; and
  - a recognition of carers and families; and
  - the integration of support services across the sectors of health, social care and education;
- that interprofessional rehabilitation puts the person who is the patient at the centre of rehabilitation policy, service delivery and practice.

7.7   Using the ICF as a way to map interprofessional rehabilitation

The core themes of this book can be brought together using the framework of the ICF (WHO, 2001). Chapter 2 provided a detailed account of the ICF and then the subsequent chapters all drew upon this information to show how the ICF can be used for that particular core theme. In Chapter 3 the framework was used to inform membership of the interprofessional team, in Chapter 4 the ICF was used to underpin our understanding of the processes of rehabilitation (assessment, goal planning, intervention and evaluation) and in Chapter 5 the domains of the ICF were used to inform choice of an outcome measure. In this chapter we use three case studies to show how the person at the centre of rehabilitation can have their rehabilitation 'mapped out' using the ICF framework.

The first case, Simon, is an example of someone for whom rehabilitation is about restoring function following a traumatic injury. The second case, Angela, is an example of a young woman with a long-term disabling condition for whom rehabilitation is about maximizing function in an ongoing situation. The final case, Mary, provides an example of the complexity of health issues arising from old age, demonstrating how the focus of rehabilitation is about maximizing independence and ability to self-care yet at the same time planning for inevitable deterioration over time.

Case study one: Simon

Simon is 29-years-old and was involved in a road traffic accident when his motorbike slid under the path of an oncoming vehicle (see Table 7.1). Simon remained conscious but his left leg was trapped in the debris from the crash. Later he underwent extensive surgery to save the leg. Wound healing was delayed due to poor blood supply to the limb and Simon had to undergo further surgery to have the leg amputated above the knee. Although the stump wound healed very well Simon complained of considerable pain and was reluctant to handle the stump or engage with his physiotherapy. Instead, he preferred to use his wheelchair to leave the hospital ward so that he could have a cigarette outside.

Six weeks later Simon is at home and due to visit the artificial limb centre. He is still complaining of pain and his general practitioner (GP) has prescribed paracetamol and tramadol. Simon has been staying inside most of the time, watching TV and playing computer games. Although he has lots of friends he has not seen many of them lately, he refuses to go out to meet them or to go and watch the football team that he used to play for. Simon had been working for a local building company but he has not been in touch with the firm since the accident.

Case study two: Angela

Angela is 23-years-old and has cerebral palsy (see Table 7.2). This was due to oxygen starvation at birth (asphyxia) and resulted in secondary epilepsy, spastic quadriplegia and dystonia (muscle tone dysfunction and abnormal, involuntary movements affecting all four limbs, trunk and neck muscles). Current family concerns relate to worsening dystonia, leading to difficulty with transfers and posture within her wheelchair.

Angela was born at term via caesarean section for failure to progress and maternal pyrexia (high temperature). She required immediate intubation because of apnoea (not breathing) and was not extubated until day two. Seizures developed within the first 24 hours. Within 4 or 5 months, it was apparent that she had cerebral palsy with signs of generalized spasticity (high muscle tone). Periodic developmental assessments did not detect significant intellectual impairment. She is non-verbal but can communicate through gesture. From about the age of 13, the principal problem has been mixed dystonia-spasticity leading to difficulty with seating. Levodopa and oral baclofen drugs have been tried and appeared to be helpful for a few months before symptoms began to worsen.

The current situation is worsening dystonia-spasticity, despite medication (oral baclofen 100 mg daily), which prevents her from being seated comfortably and she spends a lot of her day on the floor on her back. She requires full assistance with all activities of daily living. There are no significant swallowing concerns but feeding is very prolonged. Her epilepsy is very well controlled.

Her dystonia is also associated with marked sweating and increased nutritional requirements. Although it takes a long time to feed Angela she has to have five meals a day to keep her weight stable. There are no abnormal movements during sleep. Her assessment score on the Total Barry-Albright Dsytonia scale is high.

Table 7.1 Using International Classification of Functioning, Disability and Health (ICF) terminology as a mapping tool for interprofessional rehabilitation. Case study one: Simon, involved in a road traffic accident resulting in lower limb amputation.

Health condition: trauma including lower limb amputation

Body functions & structures:	Activity:	Participation:
Impairment of the lower limb due to trauma then amputation. Loss of movement range, strength, balance and stamina. Phantom limb pain **T:** Surgeons, PTs, OTs, nurses, pain specialist/psychologist **I:** Exercises to optimize muscular strength, power, co-ordination, range of movement & balance. Stump care, pain management **E:** Outcomes measured by pain and disability tools; lower limb muscle strength tests, balance, range of movement and function tests	Limitations in tasks or actions e.g. sitting, getting up from sitting; transfers, standing, walking, running and jumping **T:** PTs, OTs, exercise professional, prosthetist, family and friends **I:** Exercises task focussed but tailored to individual activity limitations. Wheelchair prescription. Limb fitting **E:** Outcomes measured by task specific functional activity tests e.g. independence in transfers/wheelchair use, prosthetic limb use, timed up and go test, other walking tests	Restrictions to involvement in social, occupational or recreational life situations e.g. household duties, work, commuting to work, sport, socializing with friends **T:** PTs, OTs, exercise professional, social worker, occupational health staff, family and friends **I:** Rehab programme to address individual participation restrictions and create opportunities to participate with the able bodied **E:** Outcomes measured by EQ-5D; SF36/ return to work/occupations/ recreational activity or increased participation time or frequency
Environmental factors:	**Personal factors:**	
Family, physical (including housing), social, occupational, attitudinal and other external contexts **T:** Family, friends, OTs, (social worker) **I:** Individually tailored programme of exercises to perform at home, housing modifications (ramps, wheelchair access, rails, wet area shower & stool), adapted vehicle **E:** Outcomes measured by overcoming barriers, decreased use of health and social services; decreased dependence on informal carers	Age, gender, coping style, social background, education, profession, past and current experiences, behaviour patterns, character, attitudes and beliefs and other internal contexts **T:** Family, friends, OTs, psychologist, pain team specialists **I:** Rehabilitation addresses some of these factors through counselling to decrease smoking and to improve coping, performance mastery/ self-efficacy and autonomy in ongoing rehab **E:** Outcomes measured by Perceived Self-Efficacy scale; Mental Health questionnaires	

OT, occupational therapist; PT, physiotherapist; SF36, Short Form Health Survey (36 questions); T, team; I, intervention; E, evaluation.

Table 7.2 Using International Classification of Functioning, Disability and Health (ICF) terminology as a mapping tool for interprofessional rehabilitation. Case study two: Angela, a young adult with cerebral palsy.

Health condition: Cerebral palsy

Body functions & structures:	Activity:	Participation:
Severe generalized muscle weakness, spasticity and dystonia	Entirely dependent on carers for all activities of daily living including transfers, mobility, and feeding. Communication through gesture and facial expression. Unable to be seated comfortably	Restrictions to involvement in social, occupational or recreational life situations e.g. schooling, higher education, leisure activities, sports, community mobility
T: Physician, PTs, OTs, nurses, family	T: SLTs, PTs, OTs, nurses, family	T: Family and friends, OTs, social worker, IT tutor/college tutors
I: trials of medication, intrathecal baclofen infusion, sleeping programme, stretching programme	I: wheelchair and seating review and prescription, carer training and support, communication devices and equipment review	I: computer training, out of home visits to community centres, exploration of day programme availability, vocational counselling
E: Outcomes – family report, dystonia and spasticity rating scales	E: Outcomes – duration of time per day spent in wheelchair; extent of successful conversations; carer burden scales	E: Outcomes – extent to which such participation occurs

Environmental factors:	Personal factors:
Family, physical, social, occupational, attitudinal and other external contexts	Age, gender, coping style, social background, education, past and current experiences, behaviour patterns, character, attitudes and beliefs, other internal contexts
T: Family, OTs, PTs, social worker, family therapist	T: SLT, counsellor, family therapist, psychologist, family and friends
I: Rehabilitation addresses these factors by individually tailoring the rehab programme involving the family as key members of the team	I: Rehabilitation to address these factors is somewhat dependent on effective communication devices, but it may be possible to improve self-confidence, decrease fear and anxiety and promote more autonomy
E: Outcomes measured by overcoming barriers, decreased use of health and social services; decreased dependence on informal carers	E: Outcome measurement dependent on communication but may include visual analogue scales for Quality of Life; Quality of Life scales

OT, occupational therapist; PT, physiotherapist; SLT, speech and language therapist; T, team; I, intervention; E, evaluation.

Case study three: Mary

Mary is 78-years-old and recently lost her husband (See Table 7.3). They had been married for nearly 50 years. Mary lives in a small bungalow in a suburb of London, she enjoys pottering around in her small garden and belongs to a local gardening society. There is a nearby corner shop and a good bus service. Mary gave up driving 10 years previously as she was always an anxious driver and preferred her husband to drive. She has two daughters, one lives nearby and has two small children, the other lives in Scotland. Her medical history includes some gynaecological surgery many years ago to repair a prolapse, however, she still experiences mixed stress and urge urinary incontinence for which she takes oxybutynin (5 mg twice a day) and wears pads. She is also overweight and suffers from low back and leg pains. These problems, plus the anxiety she had experienced with her husband, who had cancer, meant she has difficulty sleeping and sometimes gets emotionally labile (upset). Her GP had therefore prescribed zopiclone (7.5 mg one tablet at night) to help her get to sleep and lorazepam (1 mg one tablet to be taken up to two times a day as required) to help manage the episodes of anxiety.

Caring for her sick husband had taken up most of Mary's time and energy and so she initially thought she would manage alright by herself in the bungalow and was making plans for a new 'independent' life. However, after a few weeks she had a fall in the kitchen and was unable to get up; instead she crawled to the back door and was able to call for help from a neighbour. She was taken to hospital with a fracture to her left arm at the neck of the humerus. She stayed 3 nights in hospital before being discharged home with a package of community-based care and a personal alarm system. All went well initially. Her local daughter visited regularly but it was not until the second daughter visited that they began to realize that Mary's short-term memory and her walking mobility were deteriorating. The family expressed concern about Mary's ability to stay in the bungalow.

A full assessment was carried out and identified that Mary did have very poor short-term memory that was indicative of early dementia. Her weight problem was associated with high blood sugar levels requiring medication with metformin (500 mg twice a day) and would mean restrictions to her diet. Although Mary had not had any more falls she said she was worried about her balance and found walking difficult because of the pain in her legs, she complained that her legs got tired very quickly. She was particularly anxious about getting to the toilet in time and of being left on the floor again even though she had the alarm. It was not clear what was causing her low back and leg pains so a referral to orthopaedic outpatients was made, however in the interim pain medication was prescribed (paracetamol 500 mg one to two tablets up to four times a day as required *or* co-codamol (500 mg one to two tablets up to four times a day as required). The number of different medications being prescribed was also a source of worry for her daughters as they felt Mary was getting into a muddle about what to take when.

A family meeting was convened to determine what could be done to maximize Mary's ability to self-care and to lead an independent life in her bungalow, or whether the time had come for her to move into a residential care home.

For all three cases their situations have been documented in accordance with the ICF framework as depicted in Tables 7.1, 7.2 and 7.3. For such complex cases we propose that this mapping approach is a useful exercise for a rehabilitation team to employ, at least as a starting point for working interprofessionally. It ensures everyone has a shared understanding about what the rehabilitation process is aiming to

Table 7.3 Using International Classification of Functioning, Disability and Health (ICF) terminology as a mapping tool for interprofessional rehabilitation. Case study three: Mary, an older adult with complex needs.

Health condition: frail elderly person

Body functions & structures:	Activity:	Participation:
Fractured humerus. Pain. Decreased balance, leg muscle strength and endurance. Anxiety. Loss of short term memory. Loss of continence. Overweight. High blood sugar	Activities of daily living and self care. Walking. Sleeping	Restrictions to involvement in social, occupational or recreational life situations e.g. social clubs and visiting friends, church, shopping, community mobility, gardening
T: Orthopaedic/care of elderly ward team, psycho-geriatrician, psychologist, pharmacist, dietician, family	**T:** Community PTs, OTs, CPN, home carer team, GP, pharmacist, dietician, family	**T:** Family and friends, OTs, CPN
I: fracture management, medication, exercises, walking aids, dietary advice, memory aids	**I:** exercises and mobility aids, equipment and practice. Dietary advice. Memory aids and medication dispensing aids	**I:** visits to day care centre, attending church and clubs
E: Outcomes – Berg balance scale, muscle strength, shoulder ROM, leakage episodes/no of pads, memory test, pain scale, weight/BMI	**E:** Outcomes – 10 m timed walk or timed up and go; number of falls or near miss falls; medication adherence; Nottingham Activities of Daily Living scale; sleep scale	**E:** Outcomes – extent to which such participation occurs, Community Integration Questionnaire, Quality of Life scales

Environmental factors:		Personal factors:
Family, physical, social, occupational, attitudinal and other external contexts		Age, gender, coping style, social background, education, past and current experiences, behaviour patterns, character, attitudes and beliefs, other internal contexts
T: Family and friends, OTs, PTs, CPN		**T:** Psychologist, CPN, family and friends
I: Rehab programme includes: aids and equipment to enhance environmental accessibility of bungalow (internally and externally); support involvement of family		**I:** Rehabilitation to address these factors may include: counselling to improve self-confidence, decrease anxiety and assist with memory decline; support ability to self care; support in any transition to residential care
E: Outcomes measured by overcoming barriers, lack of increase in health and social services or number of hospital admissions		**E:** Outcomes measured by Perceived Self-Efficacy Scale; Beck Depression Inventory

CPN, community psychiatric nurse; GP, general practitioner; OT, occupational therapist; PT, physiotherapist; T, team; I, intervention; E, evaluation..

achieve for Angela, Mary or Simon as well as a common language to aid communication across the team. Clearly the map operates at one particular time point and so would need updating at appropriate intervals, particularly for Angela as she gets older and her condition alters or for Mary as her living circumstances change and her health deteriorates.

7.8   Revisiting the definition of rehabilitation

In considering the primary task of rehabilitation, this book has focused mainly on the idea that our domain of interest is 'functioning'. The key target of rehabilitation interventions is taken to be some aspect of 'functioning' (as described by the ICF). However, another very interesting concept that may have strong parallels with rehabilitation practice is 'capability' and 'freedom'. Siegert and colleagues have argued that restoration of human rights to people with disabilities following injury or illness can be seen as one of the objectives of rehabilitation (Siegert and Ward, 2010; Siegert et al., 2010). Using a model of human rights that has the values of 'freedom' and 'well-being' at their core these authors discuss how rehabilitation is able to restore rights that may have been lost or diminished as a result of ill-health. In a sense, human rights can be seen as a key outcome of successful rehabilitation.

There is another way to consider human rights in the context of disability. Article 27 of the Universal Declaration of Human Rights states that 'Everyone has the right freely to participate in the cultural life of the community, to enjoy the arts and to share in scientific advancement and its benefits' (United Nations, 2011). Among other human rights articulated by the Declaration, this strongly suggests that participation in ordinary community life is a fundamental human right and that exclusion is a breach of those rights. If we consider disability to be located within societal failure to accommodate to people with impairment, rather than located within individuals with impairment (the social model of disability versus the biomedical model of disability), and define disability as restrictions in community participation of differently abled people, due to barriers imposed by the way society conducts itself, then it follows that disability is actually synonymous with a breach in the human right to full community participation. This certainly does not imply that we have a right to perfect health. Disability and health can be related but are clearly not the same thing. What is implied though, is that society needs to make much more effort to minimize disability, not just to accord people with disabilities the same human rights as everyone else. This does not mean just considering environmental barriers, but includes access to rehabilitation services and technologies that aim to improve people's autonomy and participation in their communities. When rehabilitation is defined as a process that aims to accomplish these kinds of outcomes, rather than being concerned with improving impairments, then it follows that there is also a 'right to rehabilitation'.

Freedom is a concept that is clearly not limited to rehabilitation practice. Amartya Sen, the Nobel prize winning economist, has written about freedom as a key requirement and driver for economic development (Sen, 1979, 2000). But there are many parallels with his writing about freedom and what we have described in this book as good rehabilitation practice:

- success of society is measured by freedom of its members versus success of rehabilitation measured by the ability of the client to do what he/she wishes;
- health is only 'good' to the extent it allows freedoms versus better functioning is only 'good' to the extent it achieves the client's goals;
- freedom is both the 'ends and the means' versus participation as learning is as important as learning to participate.

Having made the point that disability and health are quite different things there have been recent moves to redefine health so that it better reflects the emphasis on living with chronic conditions and maximizing capacity to participate in life, given that these ongoing conditions have to be managed rather than cured (Huber et al., 2011). These authors propose that health should be defined as 'the ability to adapt and to self-manage' within the context of having capacity to manage a complex set of circumstances (Huber et al., 2011). The problem with this proposed change in definition is that there may still be the tendency to divide people into 'healthy' or 'un-healthy' categories. In reality we all have varying degrees of 'healthiness' or 'un-healthiness', or as we have already mentioned we are all disabled (or differently 'abled'), some more so than others. So although we support the need for a discussion about possible redefinitions of health we are more intrigued by how 'adaption' and 'self-management' can be defined and measured. Huber and colleagues (2011) indicate that some assessment of well-being or happiness will be needed to judge the success of a person's adaptation or self-management. In the rehabilitation setting we would emphasize the importance of partnership, between service user and provider, and that self-management arises from 'productive partnerships' that are likely to result in better health outcomes (Verkaaik et al., 2010).

The definitions we gave of rehabilitation at the start of this book did go some way to show how we are already thinking and practising with some of these concepts in mind. Thus, rehabilitation is not necessarily about returning someone to their pre-injury or pre-illness state, rather it is about helping the person to maximize their functioning within a given health condition, including a condition that may be deteriorating over time (like the case study of Angela in the preceding section). We can therefore now go on to consider some areas of healthcare where we might extend the model of rehabilitation practice.

One area of healthcare that has already been doing this is in the domain of palliative and end of life care. For example, there is an increasing awareness that rehabilitation and palliative care can learn from each other and that patients might benefit from a seamless interface between these two disciplines. Cancer treatments are now so advanced that many people with cancer are living with the illness rather than dying from it. At the same time many people with degenerative neurological conditions eventually require palliative care either at home or in a hospice or hospital. This means that patients requiring rehabilitation will often also require palliative care and sometimes both. The two fields both deal mostly with chronic and/or incurable conditions and share a focus on enhancing quality of life rather than curing a condition. Consequently, there is much for professionals to learn and potential benefits for patients and their families through increasing communication and even integration of these two disciplines (Turner-Stokes et al., 2008).

The ageing population adds further to the need for managing chronic and complex conditions. Rehabilitation professionals with limited resources have also to rethink their traditional approaches of delivering therapeutic treatments to patients and instead will need to work on ways to help patients self-manage their conditions, in much the same way as a mentor might do for helping someone in their personal development.

Finally, advances in biomedicine continue to obviate some of the needs for ongoing treatment. For example, developments in the speciality of regenerative medicine include things such as implants of stem cells that have the potential to grow into functional neurones or joint cartilage cells. These exciting developments do not mean rehabilitation is redundant; rather that rehabilitation practice will change as patients require guidance about how to train their new neurones or look after their new joint cartilages.

7.9   Limitations related to the scope of this textbook

Although we have covered a number of topics in this textbook we are not claiming this is a comprehensive guide to all rehabilitation practice. Instead, we have focused on five core themes and also recommend to interested readers that they explore further some of the ideas presented and make use of the recommended additional resources listed at the end of each chapter. For example, we suggest there is still much to be learnt from broadening our knowledge about contextual factors such as ethnic and cultural perspectives. Further examination of cultural awareness or sensitivity and cultural safety will also be helpful (Bhopal, 2006; Polaschek, 1998; Reid et al., 2000).

Other debates related to rehabilitation practice are also important. For example William Levack (personal communication, 2011) has highlighted the concern that rehabilitation planning can cause conflict within teams and distress for individual personnel (Mukherjee et al., 2009). Levack proposes that a deeper understanding of general ethical principles (e.g. Blackmer, 2000) and how they could be applied to rehabilitation planning and practice might be useful for addressing these concerns. Levack notes that many of the ethical dilemmas facing rehabilitation professionals do not relate to life and death situations (unlike much of medical ethics) so it is necessary for a more sophisticated consideration of ethics in rehabilitation practice to be developed (Levack, personal communication, 2011). For further reading on this topic see Levack (2009), Siegert and Ward (2010) and Siegert et al. (2010).

In addition we have not debated some specific areas of practice, such as the transitional care between children's services and adult services for people with disabling conditions acquired in childhood. This is becoming increasingly important as more children with severe and complex conditions survive into adulthood.

Finally, although we have briefly mentioned advances in biomedical technology as having an impact on rehabilitation practice, we have not given extensive coverage to this topic, nor to the implications arising from developments in telemedicine, internet service provision or global healthcare initiatives.

7.10   Future directions of interprofessional rehabilitation

Throughout this book we have provided examples of how research evidence informs rehabilitation practice but we specifically want to highlight here some developments in the research agenda that are likely to have a substantial impact on rehabilitation research. The first is the publication by the Medical Research Council of Great Britain of a framework for developing and evaluating complex interventions (Medical Research Council, 2008).

The Medical Research Council complex interventions framework provides opportunity for unpacking the 'black box' of rehabilitation intervention (DeJong et al., 2004). To produce the strongest evidence for the effectiveness of a treatment the recommended approach is to carry out a definitive clinical trial. For a new drug this means a double-blinded, randomized, placebo-controlled trial. Clearly this is methodologically challenging to do for many rehabilitation interventions. For example, in the context of interventions that require active engagement (e.g. exercises) on the part of the patient, it is seldom possible to blind the therapist who is providing the rehabilitation intervention and nearly always impossible to blind the patient about which intervention they are receiving. The Medical Research Council framework allows for a more pragmatic approach to trial design yet at the same time ensuring the research is carried out in as robust a manner as is possible. This is achieved by recommending an iterative process involving four stages: development (including feasibility and pilot work), evaluation (the clinical trial), dissemination, and sustainability (including implementation or return to the development stage for the next iteration to occur). Key recommendations are for the embedding of process evaluation during the work, the use of qualitative research approaches to capture the experiences of people participating in the research (patients, carers and providers), and the active involvement of patients, carers and the public in all stages of the research. These recommendations can result in detailed work to document or 'map' the intervention (see for example Abraham and Michie, 2008) to create a protocol that can be used to cross-check whether or not health professionals are delivering the intervention with fidelity to the original treatment programme.

In the example of an exercise programme the intervention map might include details of the precise techniques a therapist uses to teach strengthening exercises to a patient. The details provided are likely to include the choice of exercises, the muscle action required, the order of exercises, the number of repetitions and sets, the rest periods between sets, exercises and repetitions, the resistance used (intensity), the repetition speed and the weekly training frequency (Hoffman et al., 2005). An intervention map, like this one for an exercise programme, can then also be used to help assess whether or not the patients are adhering to the intervention. The map might also include details about the strategies used for motivating the patient to do their exercise as well as provide details about the mode of delivery (e.g. group exercise classes or an individually tailored home programme). Planning a process evaluation also ensures data are collected on recruitment rates, attrition rates and loss to follow-up as well as whether the intervention or the research process was acceptable or not. The qualitative work complements this and helps to uncover the experiences of participants and providers thereby providing further information about *why* the intervention did or did not work (as opposed to the trial, which only answers the question 'does it work?').

The Medical Research Council framework strongly recommends the involvement of service users in the development and process evaluation work. We have already introduced the concept of patient and public involvement in research as a way of demonstrating the importance of including the patient as part of a rehabilitation team (Chapter 3) and of putting the patient in the centre of rehabilitation practice (Chapter 6). Although the benefits of patient and public involvement (PPI) are yet to be fully evaluated a review has been undertaken about the impact of PPI within applied health research. The review reported that PPI helped to increase recruitment to projects, was of particular value within clinical trials and qualitative research, and was found to benefit both research participants as well as those taking part in the PPI process (INVOLVE, 2009).

As the most recent Medical Research Council framework was only updated in 2008 it is still a relatively new approach to designing clinical trials and the development work phase for interventions such as complex rehabilitation programmes can take years. So the lead-in time to the definitive trial can be quite long and a full-effectiveness and cost-effectiveness trial can take several years to complete, especially if long-term follow-up is required. Thus, the results of such research endeavours will be forthcoming sometime in the future, creating an exciting possibility that such work will help to expand the evidence base for rehabilitation practice.

A further impact of research upon rehabilitation practice that is yet to be fully appreciated is the paradigm shift concerning brain recovery processes following acquired brain injury such as stroke or trauma. A paradigm shift (see Kuhn, 1962) occurs when an accepted way of thinking is completely overtaken by new knowledge, a classic example of such a shift occurred when people realized that the Earth was not at the centre of the universe but was just another planet revolving around the Sun (see Siegert et al., 2005 for discussion of the Copernican revolution in astronomy as one of Thomas Kuhn's archetypal paradigm shifts). In acquired brain injury the traditional view was that, once damaged, the brain could not recover and there was no new growth of neurones. Instead, improvements in functional ability could only occur through compensation techniques (either other parts of the brain taking over the role of the damaged area or physical strategies involving other body parts that compensated for the lack of function in affected areas). Rehabilitation interventions and practices were orientated around this premise. More recently it has been demonstrated that new growth of brain cells, and the connections between them, can occur. This phenomena is called neuroplasticity (see Robertson, 2000) and this opens up huge possibilities for learning again how to perform functional activities. Indeed, we are all neuroplastic and have the ability to learn new things throughout our lives, albeit at probably a slower pace than when we were children. The implications for rehabilitation interventions and service provision are substantial; stroke survivors should no longer be told that their recovery has reached a 'plateau' (and so rehabilitation provision stopped). Instead, we suggest rehabilitation professionals will have to find a way of supporting patients to move on to self-training by learning how to plan, set goals and implement their own rehabilitation programmes. Research has yet to be undertaken that demonstrates such approaches are effective for long-term stroke survivors, but some services in the UK are already beginning to adopt this type of approach in the later stages of rehabilitation for people with acquired brain injury (Balchin, 2011).

In terms of the future of healthcare more generally an interesting development that is likely to have an impact on rehabilitation has arisen from the WHO's 'Framework for Action on Interprofessional Education and Collaborative Practice' (WHO, 2010). This document provides a comprehensive overview of interprofessional working, taking a global perspective and encompassing all health professions and policy makers as well as those allied to education, housing and environment. The WHO framework links interprofessional education (IPED) and communities of collaborative practice (see Chapter 3) as the future for health and education systems. The proposed framework is also regarded as addressing the demographic changes in health and well-being in the context of the increasing prevalence of chronic and complex conditions. Table 7.4 provides a summary of the mechanisms identified in

Table 7.4 Summary of identified mechanisms that shape interprofessional education and collaborative practice. (World Health Organization, 2010 reproduced with permission.)

Interprofessional education	Collaborative practice	Health and education systems
Educator mechanisms	*Institutional supports*	*Health-services delivery*
Champions	Governance models	Capital planning
Institutional support	Personnel policies	Commissioning
Managerial commitment	Shared operating procedures	Financing
Shared objectives	Structured protocols	Funding streams
Staff training	Supportive management practices	Remuneration models
Curricular mechanisms		*Patient safety*
Adult learning principles	*Working culture*	Accreditation
Assessment	Communication strategies	Professional registration
Compulsory attendance	Conflict resolution policies	Regulation
Contextual learning	Shared decision-making processes	Risk management
Learning outcomes		
Logistics and scheduling	*Environment*	
Programme content	Built environment	
	Facilities	
	Space design	

the WHO report that will shape the future of interprofessional education and collaborative practice within healthcare and education systems.

The WHO's Framework for Action indicates that there will remain a strong drive for IPED to be embedded in health professional training programmes. The challenges ahead lie in implementing this and in creating the communities of practice that underpin collaborative working. The Framework is not prescriptive as such, instead the report intends to offer ideas to 'policy-makers with ideas on how to *contextualize* their existing health system, *commit* to implementing principles of interprofessional education and collaborative practice, and *champion* the benefits of interprofessional collaboration' (WHO, 2010, p. 11). The mechanisms listed in Table 7.4 will help achieve this and are salient to rehabilitation practice regardless of the global scope and context of the original Framework report.

These ideas about the future are just that, they are possibilities rather than an attempt to predict things. However, we do believe that the five core themes presented in this book are unlikely to quickly go out of fashion and will stand you in good stead and help you adapt to the advances and changes that do occur. Nevertheless, the themes are not intended as a new dogma about how interprofessional rehabilitation should be done. Therefore, despite the evolution of professional roles, good practice in rehabilitation is likely to reflect the themes of this book, irrespective of new technologies or changing team structures. By holding on to these core values we believe that good rehabilitation practice will be maintained.

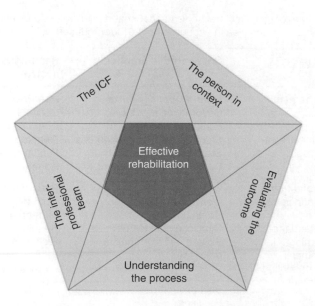

Figure 7.1   The five core themes as a framework for effective rehabilitation practice. ICF, International Classification of Functioning, Disability and Health.

7.11   Conclusion

This book has introduced you to rehabilitation through five core themes. You will have noticed that each theme is not independent, but overlaps and is strongly related to the other themes. Together, this framework forms a network of inter-connecting ideas that we believe lie at the heart of effective rehabilitation practice (see Figure 7.1).

We believe that we have laid down a challenge to you to think outside your own professional box; we are not asking you to go beyond your competencies, but rather to keep an open, enquiring mind about your practice and the role you can play in an effective interprofessional rehabilitation team. Careful reflection on your practice in the light of the core values promoted here will go a long way in helping you become an effective rehabilitation health professional.

Additional resources

Bhopal, R. (2006). Racism, socioeconomic deprivation, and health in New Zealand. *The Lancet, 367*, 1958–1959.

Levack, W. M. M. (2009). Ethics in goal planning for rehabilitation: a utilitarian perspective. *Clinical Rehabilitation, 23*(4), 345–351.

Richardson, S. (2004). Aotearoa/New Zealand nursing: from eugenics to cultural safety. *Nursing Inquiry, 11*(1), 35–42.

Sen, A. (2000). *Development as Freedom*. New York: Anchor Books.

References

Abraham, C. and Michie, S. (2008). A taxonomy of behavior change techniques used in interventions. *Health Psychology, 27*(3), 379–387.

Balchin, T. (2011). *The Successful Stroke Survivor: A New Guide to Functional Recovery from Stroke*. Lingfield: The ARNI Trust.

Blackmer, J. (2000). Ethical issues in rehabilitation medicine. *Scandinavian Journal of Rehabilitation Medicine, 32*(2), 51–55.

Bhopal, R. (2006). Racism, socioeconomic deprivation, and health in New Zealand. *The Lancet, 367*, 1958–1959.

DeJong, G., Horn, S. D., Gassaway, J., Slavin, M. D. and Dijkers, M. P. (2004). Toward a taxonomy of rehabilitation interventions: using an inductive approach to examine the "black box" of rehabilitation. *Archives of Physical Medicine & Rehabilitation, 85*(4), 678–686.

Hoffman, M. D., Sheldahl, L. M. and Kraemer, W. J. (2005). Therapeutic exercise. In: J. A. DeLisa. (Editor-in-chief). *Physical Medicine and Rehabilitation (4th edn, Vol, 1)*. Philadelphia, PA: Lippincott Williams & Wilkins.

Huber, M., Knottnerus, J.A., Green, L., van der Horst, H., Jadad, A. R., Kromhout, D., Leonard, B., Lorig K., Loureiro, M. I., van der Meer, J. W. M., Schnabel, P., Smith, R., van Wheel, C. and Smid, H. (2011). How should we define health? *British Medical Journal, 343*, d4163.

INVOLVE (2009). *Exploring Impact: Public Involvement in NHS, Public Health and Social Care Research*. London: INVOLVE.

Kuhn, T. S. (1962). *The Structure of Scientific Revolutions (2nd edn)*. London: The University of Chicago Press.

Levack , W. M. M. (2009). Ethics in goal planning for rehabilitation: a utilitarian perspective. *Clinical Rehabilitation, 23* (4), 345–351.

Medical Research Council. (2008). *Developing and Evaluating Complex Interventions: New Guidance*. London: Medical Research Council.

Mukherjee, D., Brashler, R., Savage, T. A. and Kirschner, K. L. (2009). Moral distress in rehabilitation professionals: results from a hospital ethics survey. *Physical Medicine and Rehabilitation, 1*(5), 450–458.

Polaschek, N. R. (1998). Cultural safety: a new concept in nursing people of different ethnicities. *Journal of Advanced Nursing, 27*, 452–457.

Reid, P., Robson, B. and Jones, C. P. (2000). Disparities in health: common myths and uncommon truths. *Pacific Health Dialog, 7*(1), 38–47.

Robertson, I. (2000). *Mind Sculpture*. London: Bantum Books.

Sen, A. (1979). Utilitarianism and welfarism. *The Journal of Philosophy, 76*(9), 463–89.

Sen, A. (2000). *Development as Freedom*. New York: Anchor Books.

Siegert, R. J. and Ward, A. B. (2010). Dignity, rights and capabilities in clinical rehabilitation. *Disability and Rehabilitation, 32*(25), 2138–2146.

Siegert, R. J., McPherson, K. M. and Dean, S. G. (2005). Theory development and a science of rehabilitation. *Disability and Rehabilitation, 27*(24), 1493–1501.

Siegert, R. J., Ward, T. and Playford, E. D. (2010). Human rights and rehabilitation outcomes. *Disability and Rehabilitation, 32*(12), 965–971.

Turner-Stokes, L., Sykes, N. and Silber, E., on behalf of the Guideline Development Group. (2008). Long-term neurological conditions: management at the interface between neurology, rehabilitation and palliative care. *Clinical Medicine, 8*(2), 186–191.

United Nations (2011). *The Universal Declaration of Human Rights*. New Yorks: United Nations. http://www.un.org/en/documents/udhr/ (accessed 3 December 2011).

Verkaaik, J., Sinnott, A. K., Cassidy, B., Freeman, C. and Kunowski, T. (2010). The productive partnerships framework: harnessing health consumer knowledge and autonomy to create and predict successful rehabilitation outcomes. *Disability and Rehabilitation, 32*(12), 978–85.

World Health Organization. (2001). *International Classification of Functioning, Disability and Health: ICF*. Geneva: World Health Organization.

World Health Organization. (2010). *Framework for Action on Interprofessional Education and Collaborative Practice*. Geneva: World Health Organization.

Index

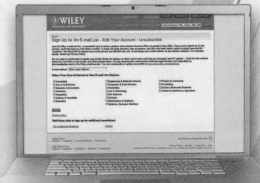
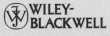